D1233110

1225

PAIN AND SUFFERING

Selected Aspects

PAIN AND SUFFERING

Selected Aspects

Edited by

BENJAMIN L. CRUE, JR., M.D.

City of Hope National Medical Center
Duarte, California
Chairman, Division of Clinical Neurology and
Director, Department of Neurosurgery;
Associate Clinical Professor of Surgery (Neurological),
University of Southern California School of Medicine, Los Angeles, California

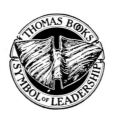

CHARLES C THOMAS · PUBLISHER
Springfield · Illinois · U.S.A.

Published and Distributed Throughout the World by

CHARLES C THOMAS • PUBLISHER

BANNERSTONE HOUSE

301-327 East Lawrence Avenue, Springfield, Illinois, U.S.A.

NATCHEZ PLANTATION HOUSE

735 North Atlantic Boulevard, Fort Lauderdale, Florida, U.S.A.

This book is protected by copyright. No part of it may be reproduced in any manner without written permission from the publisher.

© 1970, by CHARLES C THOMAS • PUBLISHER

Library of Congress Catalog Card Number: 71-111669

With THOMAS BOOKS *careful attention is given to all details of manufacturing and design. It is the Publisher's desire to present books that are satisfactory as to their physical qualities and artistic possibilities and appropriate for their particular use.* THOMAS BOOKS *will be true to those laws of quality that assure a good name and good will.*

WL 700
P 16 P
1970

LIBRARY
CORNELL UNIVERSITY
MEDICAL COLLEGE
NEW YORK CITY

JAN 2 0 1971

Printed in the United States of America

C-1

Dedicated to
Clinton H. Thienes, M.D., Ph.D.

24228 1/5/71 — 11.48

GUEST FACULTY

DONALD P. BECKER, M.D.—Chief of Neurosurgery, Harbor General Hospital, Assistant Professor of Surgery (Neurological), University of California School of Medicine, Los Angeles, California.

RICHARD BLACK, M.D.—Assistant Professor of Neurosurgery, University of Washington School of Medicine, Seattle, Washington.

KENNETH L. CASEY, M.D.—Associate Professor, Department of Physiology, University of Michigan School of Medicine, Ann Arbor, Michigan.

PETER J. JANNETTA, M.D.—Associate Professor and Chairman, Department of Neurosurgery, Louisiana State University School of Medicine, New Orleans, Louisiana.

THEODORE KURZE, M.D.—Professor of Surgery (Neurological) (Chairman), University of Southern California School of Medicine, Los Angeles, California.

BLAINE S. NASHOLD, M.D.—Division of Neurosurgery, Duke University School of Medicine, Durham, North Carolina.

FREDERICK W. PITTS, M.D.—Associate Professor of Surgery (Neurological), University of Southern California School of Medicine, Los Angeles, California.

HUBERT W. SMITH, M.D., LL.D.—Director of Interprofessional Studies, College of Law, University of Oklahoma, Norman; Consulting Psychiatrist, Department of Psychiatry and Behavioral Science, College of Medicine, University of Oklahoma, Oklahoma City; and Chancellor, The Law-Science Academy of America.

RICHARD A. STERNBACH, Ph.D.—Associate Professor of Psychiatry, University of Wisconsin School of Medicine, Madison, Wisconsin.

WILLIAM P. WILSON, M.D.—Department of Psychiatry, Duke University School of Medicine, Durham, North Carolina.

PARTICIPANTS FROM CITY OF HOPE NATIONAL MEDICAL CENTER, DUARTE, CALIFORNIA

RALPH L. BYRON, JR., M.D.—Acting Chairman, Division of Surgery, and Director, Department of Oncologic and General Surgery; Clinical Professor of Surgery, University of California, Irvine, California.

ENRIQUE J. A. CARREGAL, M.D., Ph.D.—Consultant, Department of Clinical Neurological Research; Associate Professor of Physiology, University of Southern California School of Medicine, Los Angeles, California.

BENJAMIN L. CRUE, JR., M.D.—Chairman, Division of Clinical Neurology, and Director, Department of Neurosurgery; Associate Clinical Professor of Surgery (Neurological), University of Southern California School of Medicine, Los Angeles, California.

LOUIS P. DUEMLER, M.D.—Director, Department of Medical Neurology; Assistant Clinical Professor of Neurology, University of Southern California School of Medicine, Los Angeles, California.

DAVID B. MALINE, M.D.—Senior Neurosurgeon, Department of Neurosurgery.

DANIEL V. RIIHIMAKI, M.D.—Senior Surgeon, Department of Oncology and General Surgery.

EUGENE ROBERTS, Ph.D.—Chairman, Division of Neurosciences.

SIMON RODBARD, M.D.—Director, Department of Cardiology; Associate Clinical Professor of Medicine, University of Southern California School of Medicine, Los Angeles, California.

EDWIN M. TODD, M.D.—Senior Neurosurgeon, Department of Neurosurgery; Associate Clinical Professor of Surgery (Neurological), University of Southern California School of Medicine, Los Angeles, California.

WILLIAM H. WRIGHT, M.D.—Senior Neurosurgeon, Department of Neurosurgery; Clinical Instructor in Surgery (Neurological), University of Southern California School of Medicine, Los Angeles, California.

ROBERT H. YONEMOTO, M.D.—Senior Surgeon and Associate Director, Department of Oncologic and General Surgery; Assistant Clinical Professor of Surgery, University of California, Irvine, California.

INSTITUTE FOR BIOMEDICAL STUDIES
COMMITTEE OF THE BOARD OF DIRECTORS

PERCY SOLOTOY, *Chairman;* HERMAN KRANZ, *Co-chairman;* HON. DAVID COLEMAN; ISADORE FAMILIAN; SAMUEL H. GOLTER; CHARLES HOWARD; MAURICE KANTRO; MANUEL F. ROTHBERG; LOUIS TABAK.

EMANUEL H. FINEMAN, *President*
City of Hope
BEN HOROWITZ, *Executive Director*
City of Hope

PREFACE

"Out of this potentiality for organizing complex integration there is evolved in the synaptic nervous system a functional grading of its reflex arcs and centres. Thus, with allied reflexes, the mechanism of the common path knits together by plurireceptive summation not only the separate individual stimuli of similar kind, that is tangoreceptive or photoreceptive received from some agent as this latter becomes prepotent in the environment; but it knits together separate stimuli of even wholly different receptive species." Taken from *The Integrative Action of the Nervous System* by Charles S. Sherrington, New Haven, Yale University Press, 1906.

THERE remains at present an obvious gulf between the basic neurophysiologist studying single neurone repetitive discharge in the laboratory, and the clinical electroencephalographer or neurologist interested in motor epilepsy. This chasm rapidly deepens with few bridges for communication if neurosurgeons, often frustrated by their unsuccessful treatment of patients with chronic pain syndromes in non-malignant conditions, wonder aloud about the possibility of central epileptiform activity involving the neurone aggregates in the sensory system of the human brain. This already deep canyon then widens even further as others interested in pain and suffering attempt to interject their own viewpoints—the general surgeon, anesthesiologist, internist, pharmacologist, psychiatrist, psychologist, and finally the attorney. There must be a better coordinated assault on the problem of pain if we are to develop in the near future any new integrated comprehensive concept concerning human pain and suffering. A real team effort seems to be needed. The symposium on Pain and Suffering held at the City of Hope National Medical Center, Duarte, California, on May 10, 1969, represents one such effort. This book presents the results from that symposium.

The report is neither lengthy nor comprehensive because this was a one-day meeting. It does not give an overall picture of modern pain therapy as, for example, does the monumental text, *Pain, Its Mechanisms and Neurosurgical Control,* by Drs. James White and William Sweet. Furthermore, it cannot be compared with the comprehensive reports of larger symposia on pain such as the Henry Ford Hospital International Symposium, *Pain,* edited by Drs. Robert Knight and Paul Dumke, held in Detroit in 1964; or the two-day symposium held in San Francisco in 1966 and reported as *New Concepts in Pain and Its Clinical Management,* edited by Dr. E. Lee Wong Way; or, the more recent volume entitled *Pain,* edited by Drs. A. Soulairac, J. Cahn and J. Charpentier, the report of the International Symposium on Pain organized by the Laboratory of Psychophysiology Faculty of Sciences, Paris, 1967. Furthermore, no attempt has been made to present in depth any one specific clinical problem; as, for example, the problem of trigeminal neuralgia, which had been discussed at University of California, Los Angeles, in 1966 and presented in a supplement to the *Journal of Neurosurgery,* January, 1967.

Instead, this more limited presentation is an outgrowth of certain clinical neurosurgical operative procedures attempting alleviation of pain and suffering, performed by the editor in collaboration with his present associates, Drs. Todd, Carregal, Wright and Maline, and former mentors and associates, Drs. Shelden, Pudenz and Freshwater. This includes reports on the trigeminal "compression procedure" for tic douloureux, percutaneous trigeminal tractotomy, posterior approach percutaneous high cervical chordotomy, sacral rhizotomy and compression of the intracranial portion of the seventh nerve with section of the nervus intermedius for hemifacial spasm. Also included are presentations by colleagues at the City of Hope, including Dr. Todd and Dr. Wright who discussed the technique utilizing the Todd-Wells headrest for stereotaxic hypophysectomy and thalamotomy. Incomparable data obtained from an extensive series of adrenalectomies performed by Drs. Byron, Yonemoto and Ruhimaki in the treatment of metastatic breast carcinoma are presented. Concepts concerning pain in ischemic muscle have long interested Dr. Rodbard and are discussed by him.

Invited outside faculty participants were all from the United States. Drs. Jannetta and Nashold were invited because of their recent contributions in developing new operative neurosurgical procedures for the alleviation of pain; specifically, a partial trigeminal rhizotomy under the operative microscope and stereotaxic mesencephalic tractotomy with significant neurophysiological recordings. Drs. Pitts and Kurze have had wide experience with the lateral approach for percutaneous cervical cordotomy as developed by Mullan and Rosomoff. Drs. Black and Becker were invited because of their recent contributions to a better understanding of specific portions of basic neurophysiology underlying pain syndromes. Dr. Casey, who has worked in conjunction with Dr. Melzak, has developed an excellent physiologic view of the problem of pain. Dr. Sternbach, with his recent outstanding monograph on *Pain, a Psychophysiological Analysis,* was invited to discuss pain from an overall point of view. Finally, Dr. Smith, who is familiar with the philosophical, historical and, from the legal standpoint, practical aspects of the problem of pain, suffering and mental anguish, was asked to summarize his thoughts.

The order of presentation is somewhat unusual. Instead of proceeding logically from anatomy to physiology to pathological and clinical aspects, this report starts with the more specific and limited clinical operative approaches to different pain problems that were presented in the morning session. The afternoon session was devoted to longer presentations on the basic neurophysiology of several facets. It closes with the "overview" presentations of Drs. Casey, Sternbach and Smith. It is hoped that the wide variety of subjects may make at least some chapters of interest to a number of readers and, thereby, justify their presentation in book form.

The editor would like to express his appreciation for the sponsorship of the Institute for Biomedical Studies of the City of Hope Medical Center. Gratitude is also expressed to Dr. Eugene Roberts, Chairman of the Division of Neurosciences at the City of Hope, for moderating the morning session, and to Dr. Louis Duemler, Director of the Department of Medical Neurology, for moderating the afternoon portion. Thanks are also extended to Mr. Richard Brundsvold and Mrs. Jan Gregory of the City of Hope Research Administration; Mrs. Antreen Pfau for editorial assistance; Mrs. Ruth Williams for help with the program; Mr. Syd Keith and Mr. Sol Abel for public relations; Mrs. Marian Tepe and Mrs. Denise Cox for secretarial help; Mr. Zolton Yuhasz and Mr. Kurt Smollens for medical illustrations; Mrs. Ruby Lockwood for library research; Mrs. Marge Storem, surgical scrub nurse; Mrs. Rinda Van Lennep and Miss Dorothy Terrel, X-ray technicians, Community Hospital of San Gabriel; and to Mr. Trent Wells for continued engineering help with the stereotaxic equipment. Grateful acknowledgment is also made to the editors and publishers of the *Journal of Neurosurgery, Confina Neurologica,* and the *Bulletin of the Los Angeles Neurological Societies* for permission to reproduce material and illustrations used in chapters 3, 5, 7, 8, 9 and 10. Portions of the stereotaxic work were given financial support from the Margaret Scott Stereotatic Neurosurgical Research Fund. Finally, the editor would like to thank Drs. Paul Wermer and Mel Jacobs of the City of Hope for their support, and once again to express his appreciation to all the participants in the symposium.

B.L.C.

CONTENTS

	Page
Guest Faculty	vii
Preface	xi

Chapter

1. BILATERAL ADRENALECTOMY IN PATIENTS WITH ADVANCED
BREAST CANCER
*Ralph L. Byron, Jr., Robert H. Yonemoto and
Daniel U. Riihimaki* 3

2. TECHNIQUE OF TRANSNASAL STEREOTAXIC RADIOFREQUENCY
HYPOPHYSECTOMY
*William H. Wright, Edwin M. Todd, Benjamin L. Crue, Jr.
and David B. Maline* 10

3. SACRAL RHIZOTOMY FOR PELVIC PAIN
*Benjamin L. Crue, Jr., Edwin M. Todd, William H.
Wright and David B. Maline* 20

4. PERCUTANEOUS CERVICAL CORDOTOMY—LATERAL APPROACH
Frederick W. Pitts and Theodore Kurze 25

5. POSTERIOR APPROACH FOR HIGH CERVICAL PERCUTANEOUS
RADIOFREQUENCY STEREOTAXIC CORDOTOMY
*Benjamin L. Crue, Jr., Edwin M. Todd, Enrique J. A.
Carregal, William H. Wright and David B. Maline* . . . 33

6. MICROSURGICAL RHIZOTOMY IN TRIGEMINAL NEURALGIA
Peter J. Jannetta 42

7. OBSERVATIONS ON THE PRESENT STATUS OF THE
COMPRESSION PROCEDURE IN TRIGEMINAL NEURALGIA
*Benjamin L. Crue, Jr., Edwin M. Todd and
Enrique J. A. Carregal* 47

8. COMPRESSION OF INTRACRANIAL PORTION OF FACIAL NERVE AND
SECTION OF NERVUS INTERMEDIUS FOR HEMIFACIAL SPASM
*Benjamin L. Crue, Jr., Edwin M. Todd and
Enrique J. A. Carregal* 64

9. PERCUTANEOUS RADIOFREQUENCY STEREOTAXIC TRIGEMINAL
TRACTOTOMY
*Benjamin L. Crue, Jr., Edwin M. Todd and
Enrique J. A. Carregal* 69

XV

10. STEREOTAXIC SURGERY FOR RELIEF OF PAIN AND SUFFERING
    Edwin M. Todd, Benjamin L. Crue, Jr., William H.
        Wright and David B. Maline 81
11. CENTRAL PAIN AND THE IRRITABLE MIDBRAIN
    Blaine S. Nashold, Jr. and William P. Wilson 95
12. TRIGEMINAL PAIN
    Richard Black 119
13. A NEUROPHYSIOLOGICAL EXAMINATION OF CENTRAL
        PAIN MECHANISMS
    Donald P. Becker 138
14. MUSCLE PAIN
    Simon Rodbard 154
15. SOME CURRENT VIEWS ON THE NEUROPHYSIOLOGY OF PAIN
    Kenneth L. Casey 168
16. STRATEGIES AND TACTICS IN THE TREATMENT OF PATIENTS
        WITH PAIN
    Richard A. Sternbach 176
17. SOME MEDICOLEGAL ASPECTS OF PAIN, SUFFERING AND
        MENTAL ANGUISH IN AMERICAN LAW AND CULTURE
    Hubert W. Smith 186

Index 205

PAIN AND SUFFERING

Selected Aspects

Chapter 1

BILATERAL ADRENALECTOMY IN PATIENTS WITH ADVANCED BREAST CANCER

RALPH L. BYRON, JR., ROBERT H. YONEMOTO AND DANIEL U. RIIHIMAKI

THREE percent of American women will have breast malignancy at some time in life. Of the three million who have or will have cancer of the breast, half of them will not be cured by present methods and will have recurrence, frequently associated with pain. The control of such pain poses a major problem.

Near the turn of the century, it was observed that removal of the ovaries caused improvement in advanced breast cancer in about 25 percent of the cases. The value of ablation of the ovaries then became questionable when inadequate doses of irradiation were used as a substitute for surgery.

Nathanson (15, 16) at Harvard noted that patients with advanced breast cancer responded to testosterone injections in 25 to 30 percent of the cases. This finding was soon confirmed by others. Unfortunately, there were troublesome side effects, e.g. voice change, beard, acne and increased libido.

Improvement also was observed in some patients who had been given large doses of estrogens. This unexpected result led to speculation that the hormonal effects might be mediated through the pituitary.

In 1951, Huggins (13) reported the beneficial effects of bilateral adrenalectomy in patients with advanced breast cancer. This was confirmed by others. The authors of this paper became interested in bilateral adrenalectomy in 1955 and sought to answer the question: Is it the replacement cortisone or adrenalectomy that produces the remission?

In work with laboratory animals, Biskind and Zondek (1, 2) have shown that estrogens travelling via the portal vein are removed by the liver, whereas cortisone in the portal vein is not removed by the liver.

Half of the left adrenal of selected patients was transplanted into the spleen during the bilateral adrenalectomy procedure. Thus, a portion of the adrenal was moved from the systemic to the portal circulation. This was done by removing the adrenal tissue from the patient, mincing it and then injecting it into the spleen from the medial side. The opening was closed with a fine silk stitch. One half of the adrenal tissue took sufficiently well to maintain the patient's cortisone balance. Of the patients who did not require cortisone, three showed objective improvement. One of these maintained improvement for twenty-six months. Galente *et al.* (10-12) achieved much the same result by anastomosing the left adrenal vein, which normally empties into the systemic circulation via the renal vein, to the splenic vein. He, too, found objective remissions. Dao (7-9) simply placed his potential adrenalectomy patients on maintenance cortisone before the surgery, showed that there was no response and then did the bilateral adrenalectomy with the usual objective response rate.

MATERIAL

This report is based on 463 patients who were subjected to bilateral adrenalectomies (3-6, 14, 17). The early operations were done partly through the abdomen (the left adrenal and ovaries) and partly through the flank (right adrenal). Mortality never dropped below 7 percent whether the patients were operated upon in one or two stages. Mortality dropped to 1.3 percent when both adrenals were removed through a high transverse abdominal incision.

PROCEDURE

The patient is placed in the supine position with the lumbodorsal area over the kidney lift. A bilateral subcostal incision (arched transverse) is outlined and the right half made first. After exploration of the abdomen to determine operability (if there is heavy liver involvement or extensive tumor in the adrenal fossae, the adrenalectomy is contraindicated), the incision is completed. The right adrenal is approached first. The hepatic flexure and the kidney are depressed by the assistant and the liver is retracted superiorly with a padded retractor. The posterior peritoneum and fascia are divided over the vena cava and the adrenal area parallel to and below the posterior liver margin. This permits exposure of the right adrenal, which is situated well above the kidney and in close association with the vena cava. The adrenal is mobilized by a combination of sharp and blunt dissection. The vessels are clipped with small stainless steel, silver or Vitallium clips. The right adrenal vein, which is short, comes off of the superior portion of the gland and enters the vena cava. Great care must be taken not to tear this vein because of the possibility of damage to the vena cava and severe ensuing hemorrhage. The vein is either ligated, transfixed or clipped.

The left adrenal is approached by mobilizing the spleen. The peritoneum, just lateral to the spleen, is divided and the spleen gently retracted medially and inferiorly. The adrenal gland on the left is identified in the angle between the superior pole of the kidney and the aorta. It is mobilized by sharp and blunt dissection. The left adrenal vein is

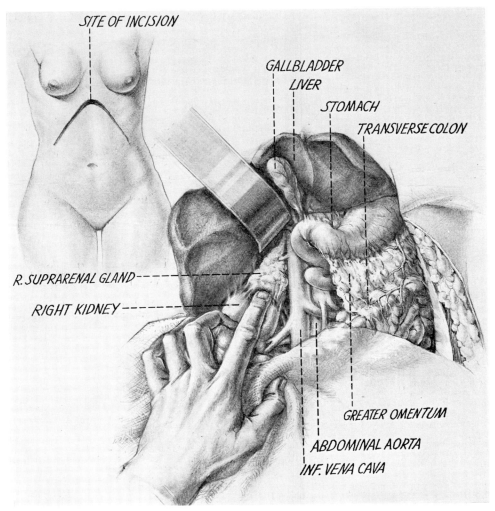

Figure 1-1. Drawing of approach to right adrenal gland.

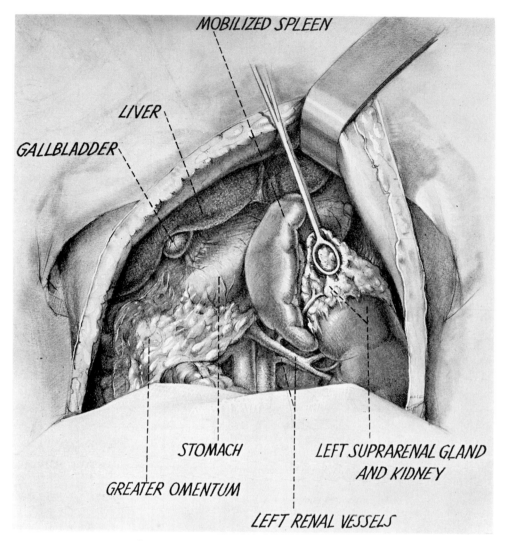

Figure 1-2. Removal of the left adrenal gland.

relatively long and arises at the junction of the lower and middle third of the gland and enters the left renal vein. It must also be ligated or clipped.

The same incision may be used to remove the ovaries. A check for uncontrolled bleeding is then made. If there is a small tear in the spleen, a piece of abdominal muscle is carefully sutured over the rent. The spleen is removed if it has extensive and deep tears.

RESULTS

Thirty-eight percent of the patients have had objective improvement which has lasted six or more months. An additional 27 percent have had subjective improvement, but measurement of visible lesions and roent-genographs have shown no regression of the neoplasms. Huggins (13) has a category for a special group of those who do not respond, i.e. neither show objective improvement or progression. About 30 percent of the patients reported in this paper might be classified this way.

It is perhaps significant that 6 percent of our patients have lived more than five years following adrenalectomy and several more than ten years. For these patients the procedure has been most worthwhile.

TABLE 1-I

RESPONSE OF PATIENTS WITH BREAST CANCER
TREATED BY BILATERAL ADRENALECTOMY

Number of Patients	463
Mortality—Last 300	1.3%
Objective Improvement	38%
Subjective Improvement	27%

In an attempt to determine when the adrenalectomy should be carried out, a randomized series was set up. Patients with extensive breast cancer which could not be treated with local surgery or irradiation were placed in the protocol. By random selection, they were treated first either with hormones or adrenalectomy. Ninety-nine patients were in the group.

TABLE 1-II

EFFECT OF ADRENALECTOMY OR HORMONES ON PATIENTS
WITH EXTENSIVE BREAST CANCER

	Adrenalectomy	Hormones
Patients (No.)	50	49
Average Duration of Improvement (Months)	20	16
Objective Improvement (Percent)	29.5	22.7
Average Survival (Months)	18	15

TABLE 1-III

Hormone Failures Having Adrenalectomy . 17 Objective Response	4 (25%)

CHEMOTHERAPY

When it is apparent that hormone manipulation is no longer beneficial, then one may consider chemotherapy. Two agents, 5-Fluorouracil and Cytoxan, have proved to be helpful in 30 to 50 percent of the cases. Cytoxan may be given intravenously—30 mg/kg loading dose and 15 mg/kg each week as long as the white blood cell count is over 4000 cu/mm. Cytoxan may also be used orally, 150 mg per day. 5-Fluorouracil may be given intravenously, 15 mg/kg at weekly intervals as long as the WBC is over 4000. It may also be given daily until symptoms of toxicity (sore mouth, depressed WBC, diarrhea, etc.) are apparent. In our hands the weekly course has been much less toxic, better tolerated and just as effective.

CONCLUSION

Bilateral adrenalectomy and/or hormone therapy appear to be of value in the management of advanced carcinoma of the breast with its prominent symptom of pain. This can be supplemented with the judicious use of chemotherapy (Cytoxan or 5-FU). The results observed by the authors suggest that bilateral adrenalectomy is somewhat more effective than hormone therapy both in frequency and duration of favorable response. The adrenalectomized patient with objective improvement requires only cortisone replacement by mouth (50 mg/day) to live a normal, productive life.

REFERENCES

1. BISKIND, M. S., and BISKIND, G. R.: Development of tumors in rat ovary after transplantation into spleen. *Proc Soc Exp Biol Med,* 55:176, 1944.
2. BISKIND, G. R., and MARK, J.: The inactivation of testosterone proprionate and estrone in rats. *Bull Hopkins Hosp,* 65:212, 1939.
3. BYRON, R. L., JR.: Bilateral adrenalectomy in advanced breast cancer (versus hormone therapy). *Chir Endocrin Cancer du Sein,* Lyon, France, May, 1966.
4. BYRON, R. L., JR.: Randomized adrenalectomies in advanced breast cancer. *Chir Endocrin Cancer du Sein,* Lyon, France, May, 1966.
5. BYRON, R. L., JR.; GREENSTONE, S., and PUZISS, I.: Bilateral adrenalectomy with splenic transplant in advanced carcinoma of the breast (abstract). *Proc Amer Ass Cancer Res,* 2:98, 1956.
6. BYRON, R. L., JR.; YONEMOTO, R. H.; BASHORE, H.; BIERMAN, H. R.; CRONEMILLER, P., and MASTERS, H.: Bilateral adrenalectomy in advanced breast cancer. *Surgery,* 52:725, 1962.
7. DAO, T. L., and HUGGINS, C.: Bilateral adrenalectomy in treatment of cancer of the breast. *Arch Surg (Chicago),* 71:645, 1955.
8. DAO, T. L., and HUGGINS, C.: Metastatic cancer of the breast treated by adrenalectomy; evaluation and the five year results. *JAMA,* 165:1793, 1957.
9. DAO, T. L.; TAN, E., and BROOKS, V.: A comparative evaluation of adrenalectomy and cortisone in the treatment of advanced mammary carcinoma. *Cancer,* 14:1259, 1961.
10. GALENTE, M.: FOURNIER, D. J., and WOOD, D. A.: Adrenalectomy for metastatic breast carcinoma. *JAMA,* 163:1011, 1957.
11. GALENTE, M., and McCORKLE, H. J.: Clinical evaluation of bilateral adrenalectomy and oophorectomy for advanced mammary carcinoma. *Amer J Surg,* 90:180, 1955.
12. GALENTE, M.; RUKES, J. M.; FORSHAM, P. H.; WOOD, D. A., and BELL, H. G.: Bilateral adrenalectomy for advanced carcinoma of the breast with preliminary observations on the effect of the liver on the metabolism of adrenal cortical steroids. *Ann Surg,* 140:502, 1954.

13. HUGGINS, C., and BERGENSTAL, D. M.: Inhibition of human mammary and prostatic cancer by adrenalectomy. *Cancer Res*, 12:134, 1952.

14. KEATING, J. L.; YONEMOTO, R. H., and BYRON, R. L., JR.: Cytotoxic drug and hormone therapy after adrenalectomy for advanced breast cancer. *Surg Gynec Obstet*, 127:538, 1968.

15. NATHANSON, I. T.: Sex hormones and castration in advanced breast carcinoma. *Radiology*, 56: 535, 1951.

16. NATHANSON, I. T.: Clinical experience with steroid hormones in breast cancer. *Cancer*, 5:754, 1952.

17. YONEMOTO, R. H.; BYRON, R. L., JR., and KEATING, J. L.: Long term survival after adrenalectomy for advanced breast cancer. *Cancer*, 20:254, 1967.

Chapter 2

TECHNIQUE OF TRANSNASAL STEREOTAXIC RADIOFREQUENCY HYPOPHYSECTOMY

WILLIAM H. WRIGHT, EDWIN M. TODD, BENJAMIN L. CRUE, JR.
AND DAVID B. MALINE

S URGICAL ablation of the hypophysis has undergone rapid advances since early attempts were reported in the 1950's (5, 6, 12, 14). In 1956, Haagensen (8) recommended that neither adrenalectomy nor hypophysectomy be considered in the treatment of a patient with metastatic breast cancer "until all other methods had failed," because of the magnitude and questionable value of the procedures at that time.

Sufficient data had been compiled by 1961 (16, 17) to establish that both procedures could produce objective response in about one-third of the patients treated, with patients in the responsive group averaging fifteen months longer postoperative survival than the nonresponders. Which procedure, then, is the procedure of choice?

Numerous investigators (4, 11, 13, 24, 25) relate continued success with various techniques of hypophysectomy; and, though there are definite theoretical advantages (7, 9, 15) to hypophysectomy over adrenalectomy, some recent reports on the management of patients with advanced breast cancer suggest that adrenalectomy has "won out" over other forms of surgical ablation (3, 18). Still others feel that the choice of the procedure should depend mainly on the skills and facilities available to the patient (26).

Avoiding the debate concerning statistical analysis of response rates (1, 16, 17) and conceding the approximately equal effectiveness of hypophysectomy and adrenalectomy, the authors believe that the technique for hypophysectomy described in this paper avoids neurologic complication, approaches completeness of removal and allows the added factors of comfort, shortened operative time, ease of management and reduction of in-hospital time, making it the procedure of choice in ablative endocrine surgery.

Talairach first reported stereotaxic transnasal hypophysectomy in 1956, and, in 1962, the results of 135 cases treated with yttrium 90 (28). Rand (19-21), in 1964, introduced a cryosurgical technique for destruction of pituitary tissue, employing a stereotaxic unit especially designed for this approach. Zervas (31), using Talairach's method but producing destruction of the gland with radiofrequency, reported his technique in

10

1965 and the results of his first sixty-five patients in November of 1967 (32).

The authors' experience with stereotaxic hypophysectomy began in mid-1964, using a cryoprobe in the manner prescribed by Rand. Four lesions effected at temperatures of –170°C to –185°C for ten to fifteen minutes for each lesion are required in order to completely destroy the normal pituitary gland with the cryoprobe (22). Earlier, six such lesions, requiring one and one-half hours for lesion-making alone, not counting cooling or heating times, were employed for hypophysectomy. Several of the early cases required six to seven hours of operating time. The shortest time was four hours, using the large probe. It was obviously mandatory to shorten the operative time.

A more versatile Todd-Wells head holder, designed to accommodate a system of preset x-ray tubes (29), greatly expedited the procedure. Operative time was shortened dramatically by replacing the cryoprobe with a radiofrequency unit for the production of lesions.

Special precautions are taken to prevent infection. The patient's hair is shampooed with hexachlorophene soap on two successive evenings prior to surgery. The nasal passages are irrigated every six hours with 2 drops of 1000 units per cc bacitracin solution and 2 drops of ¼% Neo-Synephrine® solution two days prior to surgery. At the time of surgery, the patient's nasal passages are thoroughly swabbed with cottonoids and soaked in bacitracin and Neo-Synephrine. Postoperatively, the patients are given prophylactic antibiotics for four days.

Special x-ray procedures prior to hypophysectomy have not been employed even though anatomical variation in the pituitary gland (2) is acknowledged. One patient who was not accepted for this procedure because of proximity of the carotid arteries, as demonstrated by preoperative angiography, was later successfully treated with cryohypophysectomy after a total extracapsular procedure had been abandoned. It may be that newer simplified techniques of cavernous sinus venography may facilitate more accurate placement of the probes (10, 23, 27).

Originally all patients were awake, with transtracheal block and intubation during the hypophysectomy, but they are now given general anesthesia without constant monitoring of extraocular movements or visual fields. Extraocular palsies and field defects are complications infrequently reported when lesions are made with heat or cold. These have usually been transient in nature when reported. In normal gland, where the probe is maintained within the confines of the sella, there does not appear to be any permanent damage to the chiasm or adjacent cranial nerves. This finding agrees with that recently reported by Zervas (33).

The patient's head is fixed securely in the Todd-Wells head unit,

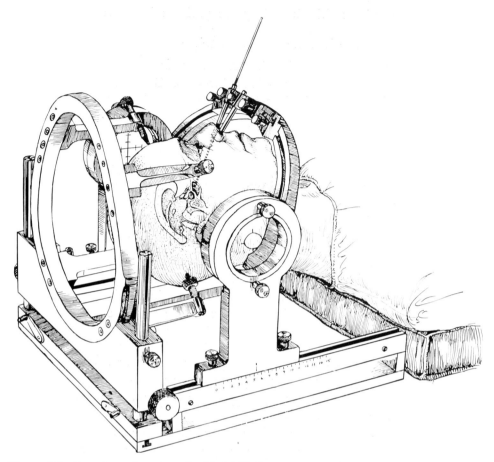

Figure 2-1. Drawing of patient in Todd-Wells stereotaxic frame positioned for transnasal hypophysectomy.

which has been columnated previously (Fig. 2-1). Preliminary films are
taken, and usually one adjustment brings the sella in the midline on the
AP and within the ring and cross hairs on the lateral view. The nasal
passages are prepared and the drill guides placed in each nostril onto the
floor of the sphenoid sinus while the preliminary films are being taken.
The mucous membrane can be injected with Xylocaine and epinephrine
to reduce the amount of bleeding and to lessen the amount of general
anesthetic required.

   Drills with an external diameter of 2.7 mm are twisted by hand
through the sphenoid sinus through the floor of the sella along a pathway
toward a predetermined point 2 mm below the tip of the dorsal sella and
2 mm from the midline, the angles of the approach varying with the con-
tour of the sella. Bilateral holes are made, and symmetrical positioning of

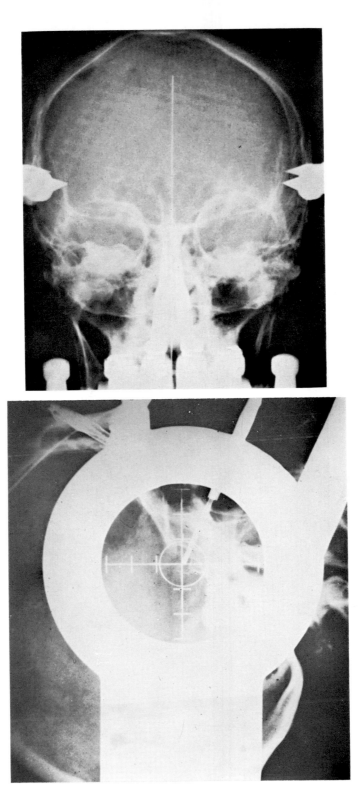

Figure 2-2. X-ray view of bilateral sleeves in place. *Top:* AP view—shows bilateral drills. *Bottom:* Lateral view—shows single probe in center of gland.

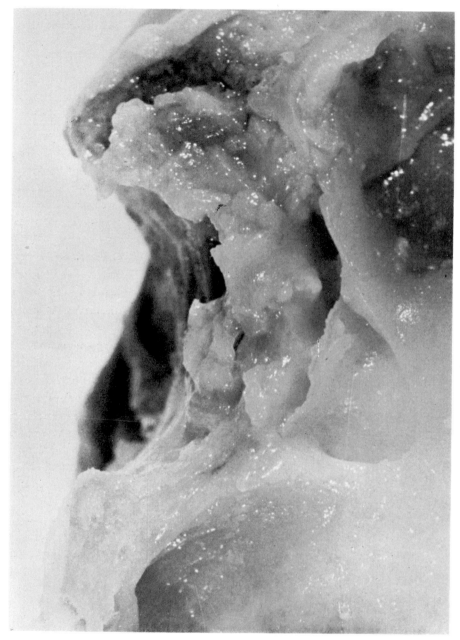

Figure 2.3. Photograph of gross specimen showing postoperative empty sella in medial cross section after three lesions on each side. (From Methodist Hospital of Southern California.)

the drills is checked by x-ray Polaroid films prior to inserting the probe. A 2.1 mm diameter probe with a 5 mm tip, containing a thermistor, is then inserted to the predetermined point at the posterior wall of the sella (Figs. 2-2A & 2-2B). Because of proximity of the diaphragm sella at this point, the 80° lesion is limited to two minutes. This prevents injury to the stalk or hypothalamus and reduces the frequency of diabetes insipidus. Wilson (30) has suggested similar modifications of freezing parameters of the cryoprobe in attempting to reduce the incidence of this complication. Three lesions are usually required on each side, with the middle and anterior inferior lesions being made at 80° for four minutes. Probes are removed as soon as the temperature at the tip reaches body temperature. Muscle concurrently removed from the patient's thigh is fragmented and inserted through a special tube designed for this purpose. Plugging the defect in the wall of the anterior sella prevents rhinorrhea. Temporary cottonoid pledgets soaked in Neo-Synephrine may be used to control any persistent bleeding from the nasopharynx.

Figure 2-3 shows a midline sagittal section from a patient who had six lesions as described above. There is no viable pituitary tissue. Figure 2-4A is a cross section of a pituitary gland from a patient who had only two lesions generated in the midline at 80°C for four minutes. A small rim of viable tissue is evident. This is shown microscopically in Figure 2-4B. The data indicate that six radiofrequency lesions are necessary to produce total destruction of the pituitary gland.

Utilizing the technique as outlined above, total operative time has been reduced to about an hour and a half. The use of general anesthesia has made this a comfortable and acceptable procedure for the patient. In our experience, this has not resulted in neurologic complications, which is in agreement with Zervas, who also employs general anesthesia (33, 34). Patients usually enjoy an evening meal and can be ambulated the following day. Rhinorrhea has not been a problem (32) with the routine use of muscle plugs. Diabetes insipidus is usually transient and can be controlled at night by the use of Pitressin. If the condition should persist, continued therapy at home is indicated and pituitary extract insufflation is used. Cortisone is administered orally (25-50 mg per day) and thyroid is initiated at about four weeks. Salt balance, especially in periods of stress, is not a concern. This is in contrast to the condition seen in adrenalectomized patients.

Our purpose has been to describe a technique of hypophysectomy by a simple, direct transnasal approach. This circumvents the formidable obstacles of open craniotomy. The advantages of stereotaxic hypophysectomy, for example the ease of surgery and postoperative management

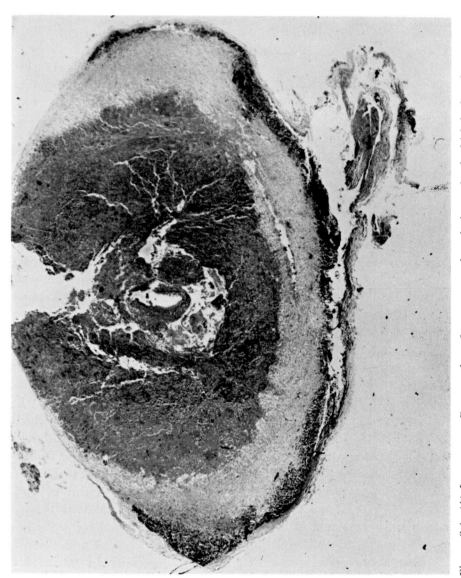

Figure 2-4. (A) Low power. Cross section of a postoperative pituitary gland which had undergone two radiofrequency lesions on each side showing outer rim of preserved or regenerating cells. (From City of Hope.)

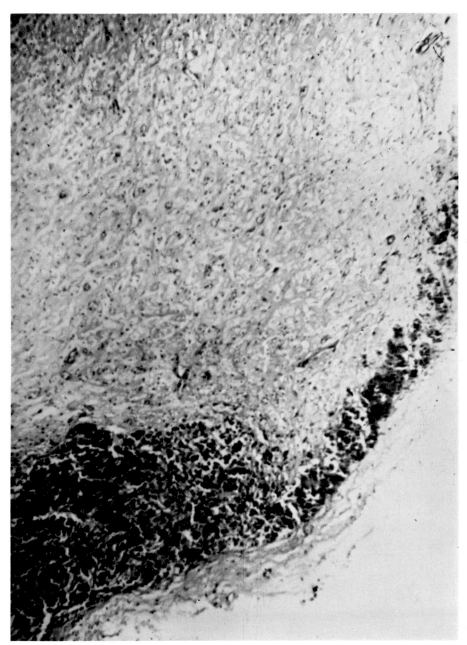

Figure 2-4. (B) High power at edge.

coupled with low morbidity, effectively repudiate the classical arguments against pituitary ablation.

REFERENCES

1. ATKINS, H.: Comparison of adrenalectomy and oophorectomy with hypophysectomy in the treatment of advanced cancer of the breast. *Proc Roy Med,* 53:638, 1960.
2. BERGLAND, R. M.; RAY, B. S., and TORACK, R. M.: Anatomical variations in the pituitary gland and adjacent structures in 225 human autopsy cases. *J Neurosurg,* 28:93, 1968.
3. CROWLEY, L. G.: Current status of the management of patients with endocrine-sensitive tumors. *Calif Med,* 110:43, 1969.
4. DIEMATH, H. E.: Zur neurochirurgieschen schmerzbekampfung bei malignomen. Chordotomien, hyperphysektomien. *Wien Klin Wschr,* 78:309, 1966.
5. FRESHWATER, D. B.; CRUE, B. L.; SHELDEN, C. H., and PUDENZ, R. H.: A technique for hypophysectomy. *Calif Med,* 84:229, 1956.
6. FRESHWATER, D. B.; CRUE, B. L.; SHELDEN, C. H., and PUDENZ, R. H.: Further experience with a technique of total extracapsular hypophysectomy. *Cancer,* 10:105, 1957.
7. FURTH, J.: Experimental foundations and practice of hormonal control of breast cancer. *Bull NY Med,* 41:509, 1966.
8. HAAGENSEN, C. D.: *Diseases of the Breast.* Philadelphia, Saunders, 1956.
9. HAHN, Do-WON, and TURNER, C. W.: Effects of ovariectomy-hypophysectomy-adrenalectomy and ovariectomy-hypophysectomy on feed intake and mammary gland growth as measured by DNA. *Proc Soc Exp Biol Med,* 126:476, 1967.
10. HANAFEE, W. N.; ROSEN, L. M.; WEIDNER, J. W., and WILSON, G. N.: Venography of the cavernous sinus, orbital veins, and basal venous plexus. *Radiology,* 84:751, 1965.
11. HARROLD, B. P.; CATES, J. E., and JAMES, J. A.: Treatment of advanced breast cancer by trans-sphenoidal hypophysectomy. *Brit J Cancer,* 22:19, 1968.
12. JESSIMAN, A. G.; MATSON, D. D., and MOORE, F. D.: Hypophysectomy in the treatment of breast cancer. *New Eng J Med,* 261:1199, 1959.
13. KENNEDY, B. J., and FRENCH, L.: Hypophysectomy in advanced breast cancer. *Amer J Surg,* 110:411, 1965.
14. LUFT, R., and OLIVECRONA, H.: Experiences with hypophysectomy in man. *J Neurosurg,* 10:301, 1953.
15. LYONS, W. R.; HAO LI, C.; AHMAD, N., and RICE-WRAY, E.: Mammotrophic effects of human hypophysial growth hormone preparations in animals and man. *Excerpta Medica,* 1968, ICS No. 158.
16. MACDONALD, I.: Adrenalectomy and hypophysectomy in disseminated mammary carcinoma. *JAMA,* 175:787, 1961.
17. MACDONALD, I.: Endocrine ablation in disseminated mammary carcinoma. *Surg Gynec Obstet,* 115:215,1962.
18. MOORE, F. D.; WOODROW, W. I.; ALIAPOULIOS, M. A., and WILSON, R. E.: Carcinoma of the breast (concluded). *New Eng J Med,* 277:460, 1967.
19. RAND, R. W.: Stereotactic trans-sphenoidal cryohypophysectomy. *Bull Los Angeles Neurol Soc,* 29:40, 1964.
20. RAND, R. W.: Stereotactic trans-sphenoidal cryohypophysectomy. *Western J Surg,* 72:142, 1964.

21. RAND, R. W., *et al.*: Stereotactic cryohypophysectomy. *JAMA*, 189:255, 1964.
22. RAND, R. W.: Cryogenic techniques in stereotaxic neurosurgery—Cryohypophysectomy and cryothalamectomy. *Int Surg*, 49:212, 1968.
23. RAND, R. W., and HANAFEE, W. N.: Cavernous sinus venography and stereotaxic cryohypophysectomy. *J Neurosurg*, 26:521, 1967.
24. RAY, B. S.: Current cancer concepts: Hypophysectomy as palliative treatment for disseminated carcinoma. *JAMA*, 200:974, 1967.
25. RAY, B. S.: Intracranial hypophysectomy. *J Neurosurg*, 28:180, 1968.
26. SEDGWICK, C. E., and VERNON, J. K.: Management of carcinoma of the breast. *Surg Clin N Amer*, 47:3, 1967.
27. TAKAKU, A., and SUZUKI, J.: A new method of orbital and cavernous sinus venography. *J Neurosurg*, 30:200, 1969.
28. TALAIRACH, J.; SZIKLA, G.; TOURNOUX, P. B., and BANCAUD, J.: La chirurgie stereotaxique hypophysaire. *Confin Neurol*, 22:204, 1962.
29. TODD, E. M., and CRUE, B. L.: An image enlargement scale for stereotactic surgery. *Amer J Roentgen*, 105:270, 1969.
30. WILSON, C. B.; WINTERNITZ, W. W.; BERTAN, V., and SIZEMORE, G.: Stereotaxic cryosurgery of the pituitary gland in carcinoma of the breast and other disorders. *JAMA*, 198:119, 1966.
31. ZERVAS, N. T.: Technique of radiofrequency hypophysectomy. *Confin Neurol*, 26:157, 1965.
32. ZERVAS, N. T., and GORDY, P. D.: Radiofrequency hypophysectomy for metastatic breast and prostatic carcinoma. *Surg Clin N Amer*, 47:5, 1967.
33. ZERVAS, N. T., and GORDY, P. D.: Radiofrequency thermal hypophysectomy. Technical note. *J Neurosurg*, 30:511, 1969.
34. ZERVAS, N. T.: Personal communication, 1966.

Chapter 3

SACRAL RHIZOTOMY FOR PELVIC PAIN

BENJAMIN L. CRUE, JR., EDWIN M. TODD, WILLIAM H. WRIGHT
AND DAVID B. MALINE

A T the present time there remains a place for open surgical sacral rhizotomy in patients suffering from pelvic pain due to uncontrolled malignant disease, in spite of recent advances in drug therapy and percutaneous pain-relieving procedures.

Midline pelvic pain has often been difficult to control by cordotomy. With open thoracic cordotomy a bilateral procedure is usually needed, requiring two operations. There is a significantly increased risk of loss of ambulation and/or urinary bladder control if this is done in one stage. The phenomenon of "sacral sparing" and unsatisfactory relief from pain is well recognized. The technique of alcohol or Pantopaque and phenol subarachnoid injection also includes some risk if significant analgesia is to be obtained. Unfortunately, with these chemical agents even the good results are often only temporary. Percutaneous cordotomy is at present done most often at the C1-C2 level and carries an added risk—possible paresis of an upper extremity and possible respiratory difficulty. Furthermore, even with an excellent immediate result from percutaneous cordotomy, long-term studies show a significant recurrence of pain if the patient survives a sufficient period of time. In many patients with sacral pain, even from malignant invasion, a prolonged clinical course is not uncommon.

Therefore, in a small selected group of patients with sacral or perineal pain resulting from proven neoplastic disease the authors have continued to perform open sacral rhizotomy, utilizing the operative procedure described previously in 1964 (1).

The patient is placed prone or on his side. His legs are wrapped with elastic bandages and the back is flexed, prepared and draped. The usual posterior approach is made through a midline lumbosacral incision. The overhanging tip of the L5 spine and the entire small S1 spine, together with the upper edge of the sacrum, are rongeured away (Fig. 3-1). The ligamentum flavum is excised, the operative defect is enlarged and the S1 and S2 roots are located. Two heavy silk ligatures are passed extradurally with a right-angle clamp. The upper ligature is tied very tightly below the axillae of the S1 roots. The second ligature is tied as far

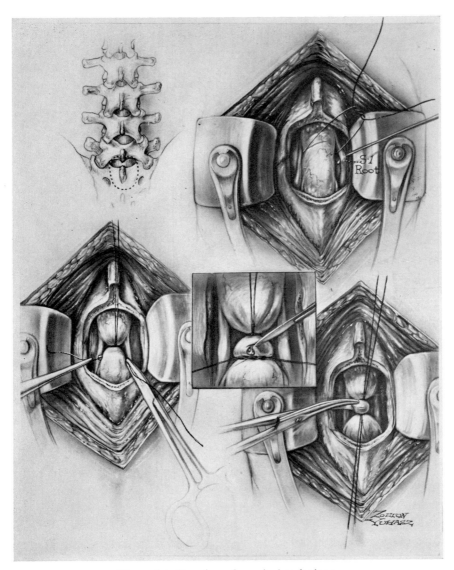

Figure 3-1. Drawing of surgical technique.

was very vascular. Excessive bleeding was frightening when the nerve was punctures the fluid-filled sac between the ligatures (Fig. 3-1, insert). This is an important minor technical point, allowing the second ligature to be tied tightly also. Then the dural sac with all of its contents is divided between the ties. (If the ligatures are not tied correctly the nerve roots will retract and the sutures will slip off the severed dural end.) The spinal canal is packed with Gelfoam or Oxycell as needed for hemostasis and the incision is closed in layers.

During the last twelve years this type of sacral rhizotomy has been performed on eighteen patients at the U. S. Naval Hospital, San Diego; the City of Hope Medical Center, Duarte; the Huntington Memorial Hospital, Pasadena; the San Gabriel Community Hospital, San Gabriel; the Southern California Methodist Hospital, Arcadia; and the Los Angeles County General Hospital, Los Angeles. The pathological diagnosis of primary malignant neoplasm was verified histologically in all eighteen cases. At the time of rhizotomy, uncontrolled metastatic disease or invasive malignancy was verified by biopsy or by roentgen-ray evidence in thirteen patients. In five cases the intractable pain was attributed to recurrent tumor rather than postoperative or postirradiation inflammation, but this was only a clinical impression prior to rhizotomy. In two of these cases epidural carcinoma was found by biopsy of the lower sacrum through the operative incision at the time of rhizotomy.

The primary tumor sites in these cases were rectosigmoid colon (10 cases), anus (1 case), cloacal carcinoma (1 case), cervix (3 cases), bladder (1 case), vulva (1 case) and one case of primary liposarcoma of the perineum.

Prior to rhizotomy, seventeen of the eighteen patients had functioning colostomies and ten had either an ileal urinary bladder or long-standing drainage by urethral catheter. All were reasonably good surgical risks and had a reasonable life expectancy. All patients were on large doses of narcotics. All were ambulatory. In all cases attempts at surgical cure had been exhausted and cobalt irradiation and chemotherapy (including intra-arterial when indicated) had also been utilized or considered not to be indicated. In addition, all of these eighteen patients had been found to have had insufficient alleviation of their suffering by available conservative methods including sedation, antidepressants (Elavil), oral analgesics or narcotics (Percodan) and strong reassurance and psychotherapeutic support.

None of the eighteen patients suffered operative mortality. There was, of course, some operative morbidity. Three patients had so much post-irradiation scarring and vascular change in the epidural space that sufficient operative hemorrhage was encountered (with known malignant disease and borderline preoperative anemia) to indicate blood transfusions during surgery. There were two postoperative wound hematomas requiring needle aspiration (no drains were used), but there were no wound infections. There were several patients who had considerable postoperative new and sometimes severe radiating sciatic pain into the buttocks and posterior thighs. While alarming to the patients, these pains subsided promptly. Surprising, perhaps, was the finding that early ambulation did not make the local back or sciatic pain worse, and only caused headache in the first few cases in which test preoperative spinal anesthesia had been done or in which the spinal fluid had been allowed to escape at the time of rhizotomy. There were no reported serious long-term dysesthesias or burning pains in the anesthetic perineum or in the lower extremities, except for the one patient reported as a failure.

Of the eighteen patients, one was listed as a failure. There were two poor results, two fair results and thirteen satisfactory results. The failure case was in a woman with carcinoma of the rectum. Postoperatively she continued to have a deep pelvic pain described as a "hot mass." This was made worse by ambulation and was not alleviated by narcotics or subsequent bilateral high thoracic open cordotomy. Tranquilizers gave her relief. (She is described in a previous report [1].)

There were two patients who had poor responses. Both had unilateral sciatic pain as well as perineal pelvic pain preoperatively, and had insufficient relief of the sciatic pain component following the surgery. One subsequently underwent cordotomy with resultant relief.

Two other patients had a preoperative sciatic pain component that was relieved by rhizotomy but in which, within a few months, severe sciatic pain recurred. They are classified as having only a fair result.

In the remaining thirteen cases there has been satisfactory long-term relief from pain. The small area of perineal and perianal anesthesia has been well tolerated. In all but the one failure case there was immediate relief from all deep pelvic pain, including the patient with spread posteriorly from the vulva.

Since previously reporting our first eight cases there have been two definite changes in our concept concerning patient selection.

First: The complaint of sciatic pain radiation preoperatively, as might have been expected, has proven to be a definite limiting factor in prognosticating adequate relief from pain by means of this procedure. Even when there has been no clinical (ankle jerk preserved) or EMG evidence of sacral plexus involvement above S2, and even when the S1 root is severed at surgery on the painful side, there has been continued or promptly recurrent postoperative sciatic pain in approximately one half of those cases in which there was a significant degree of severe preoperative pain in a lower extremity. The four poor and fair results fall in this group. This pain becomes subjectively very distressing to the patient postoperatively in spite of the cessation of the pelvic pain component. There is no question but that in our enthusiasm we unwisely tried to extend the useful limits of this procedure in this small group of patients. In the future, this type of sacral rhizotomy will not be employed except for alleviation of pelvic pain in those patients with an absent or very minimal sciatic pain component.

Second: On the contrary, the problem of postoperative paralysis of bladder and bowel control has been less of a concern than had been anticipated. The paralysis of the rectal sphincter was well accepted psychologically by the single patient without a colostomy, and the bowel problem was handled adequately by diet. In seven of the patients there had been adequate preoperative voluntary urinary bladder control. In these cases the S2 root was preserved on the less painful side, with the S2 and, at times, the S1 root severed on the most painful side. In all patients, both male and female, there was prompt return of adequate voluntary urinary bladder function and control. Thus, at the present time, with proven malignancy and uncontrolled severe pelvic pain, the presence of functioning bowel and bladder control would no longer be considered a contraindication to this type of sacral rhizotomy in an understanding, cooperative patient.

Finally, a word about postoperative cutaneous anesthesia. In view of the effective relief from pelvic pain and the grossly large number of nerve fibers cut at rhizotomy, it is surprising how small an area of perineal and perianal anesthesia can be demonstrated by pinprick test postoperatively, especially on the side where an S2 root has been spared for bladder control. It is hoped that in the future this type of patient undergoing sacral rhizotomy may be better studied pre- and postoperatively to determine the physiology of both the motor and sensory function of these sacral roots.

REFERENCE

1. CRUE, B. L., and TODD, E. M.: A simplified technique of sacral rhizotomy for pelvic pain. *J Neurosurg,* 21:835, 1964.

Chapter 4

PERCUTANEOUS CERVICAL CORDOTOMY
Lateral Approach

FREDERICK W. PITTS AND THEODORE KURZE

A NTEROLATERAL cordotomy for relief of intractable pain has been an important part of the neurosurgeon's armamentarium since its introduction by Spiller and Martin in 1912 (12). Its subsequent development by Frazier and others still continues (1, 3, 5, 9). Cordotomy performed percutaneously has extended the availability of this type of pain relief to patients incapable of withstanding a major surgical procedure. Mullan, in 1963, initially reported percutaneous cordotomy using a strontium-tipped needle (7). Many subsequent modifications have been reported by Mullan, Rosomoff and others regarding both lesion production and approach (2, 6, 8, 10). Our experience has been limited to the lateral approach and creation of lesions by radiofrequency current.

TECHNIQUE

Our technique represents a modification of the Rosomoff method (10). Premedication and subsequent supplemental medication is supervised by an anesthesiologist so that the patient can be comfortable but cooperative. The patient is placed on the x-ray fluoroscopic table supine. The head is secured by pin fixation in the Rand-Wells head rest after the scalp has been cleansed. AP fluoroscopy with image intensification is used to demonstrate the odontoid process, and lateral x-rays are taken to show the C1-C2 interspace prior to final tightening of the pins. When satisfactory position has been obtained, the area of and around the mastoid process is prepared and a lateral x-ray is taken with a localizer rod in place to indicate the optimal area for needle puncture. The skin is then infiltrated with local anesthesia, and a #18 thin-wall (TW) short-bevel needle is introduced and guided toward the anterior one-third of the spinal canal at the C1-C2 level. Usually, one lateral x-ray is taken to verify position and then the dura is punctured. The procedure is continued if the CSF is clear, but if bloody CSF is encountered the procedure is stopped since this might mitigate against the use of Pantopaque. The micromanipulator is next attached to the needle. AP fluoroscopy then demonstrates the needle tip, which is adjusted to lay just lateral to the margin of the odontoid process. Ten cc of air is next injected and then

25

1 cc of Pantopaque. A lateral x-ray is taken to demonstrate the relationship of needle to anterior cord and dentate ligament. The needle is adjusted appropriately so that the tip is directed just anterior to the dentate. The stylet is next removed and replaced with the electrode. The
authors have used 0.02 in stainless steel wire, Teflon insulated, with a
2 mm uninsulated tip. The electrode is prepared preoperatively so that
the insulation projects 2 mm beyond the midpoint of the needle bevel.
The electrode is secured in a clamp so that it cannot be advanced further
than 2 mm when being introduced. Once the electrode has been introduced through the #18 needle, the needle-electrode assembly is attached
to the RF unit, with the active cable going to the electrode and the indifferent cable to the needle shank. The needle-electrode assembly is
then advanced millimeter by millimeter while impedance is tested. When
the cord is punctured there is a marked increase in impedance. An AP
fluoroscopic view is then taken to visualize the needle tip. If it is beyond
midline of the spinal canal it is withdrawn until just medial to the
odontoid border before any lesions are created. Repetitive pulses of stimulation of 10-60/sec at about 0.5-1.0 volts are applied. The procedure is
discontinued if there is ipsilateral upper or lower extremity motor activity or failure to obtain contralateral sensory phenomena. If contralateral tingling or paresthesia occurs, a lesion is then made. The lesion is
created with a 100 ma current initially for 10 seconds. Duration of lesion
generation is then increased until the appropriate sensory level is obtained, at which time two more similar lesions are made to solidify the
effect. Should the lesion generation be unduly uncomfortable to the patient, the ma is decreased and a longer time interval is used. Throughout the procedure the patient is tested for sensory and motor function.
Upon completion of the procedure the patient is returned to his bed and
kept supine for twenty-four hours to minimize any postspinal headache.

DEMOGRAPHY

Eighty-three patients have undergone 121 procedures. These data are
summarized in Table 4-I. Indication for employment of the procedure

TABLE 4-I

DISTRIBUTION OF CORDOTOMY PATIENTS AND PROCEDURES

	Patients (number)	Primary Procedure (number)	Repeat Procedure (number)	Procedures (total)
Unilateral cordotomy	70	70	21	91
Bilateral cordotomy	13	26	4	30
Total patients	83		Total cordotomies	121

was pain caused by malignancy in fifty-nine patients and for benign causes in twenty-four. These benign causes were primarily pain secondary to multiple surgical procedures on the lumbar spine. Two were for pain from diabetic neuropathy and two for pain secondary to peripheral vascular disease. Fifteen patients had repeat procedures. These were all in our early experience with the operation.

RESULTS

There was no mortality associated with the lateral cordotomy procedure. Results have been evaluated in several ways and are summarized in Table 4-II. The sensory level as such has not been recorded separately because all of those who had beneficial results had excellent sensory levels while those considered to have had fair results had hypalgesia, but not analgesia. Three of those classified as "poor results" have excellent sensory levels but are considered poor results because of painful dysesthesia. Complications (Table 4-III) have been less than those reported following surgical cordotomy techniques (4, 11), and probably reflect upon the advantage of working with an alert cooperative patient. We have not had any apneusic respiratory complications. No bladder complications were seen in any unilateral procedures. Transient use of catheter was required with bilateral cordotomies. Patients with preexisting incontinence or bladder involvement could not be evaluated.

TABLE 4-II

RESULTS OF PERCUTANEOUS CORDOTOMY

Evaluation	Procedure (number)	Patients (number)
Good	74 (61%)	60 (72%)
Fair	9	10
Poor	38	13
Total	121	83

TABLE 4-III

COMPLICATIONS FOLLOWING PERCUTANEOUS CERVICAL CORDOTOMY

Complications*		Complication Rate	
Dysesthesia	5	Procedure	8.2% (10/121)
Hemiplegia	4	Patients	12% (10/83)
Coronary	1		

* No respiratory or bladder complications, see discussion.

DISCUSSION

The initial technique was essentially that described by Rosomoff (10). This has been modified subsequently to include pin fixation of the head, and cord visualization by both air and Pantopaque. One problem encountered was uncertainty regarding puncture of the cord, despite radiographically satisfactory needle position. Lateral cord movement has been observed by radiographic means (Fig. 4-1). This was thought to be due to a tough pia. One method that eased pial puncture was placing a sharp #22 gauge needle through the #18 TW after the latter had been advanced to touch the cord. The sharp needle punctured the pia and then was replaced with the electrode. This technique, however, has been supplanted by impedance measurements. The needle is now advanced until marked increase in electrical impedance is noted. This is indicative of cord puncture. The authors have not been concerned about pushing the cord beyond the midline if necessary to puncture the pia. No lesion is made, however, until the electrode is retracted back to the position of the ipsilateral border of the odontoid. Electrode placement within the cord, no matter how well verified by impedance measurements and radio-

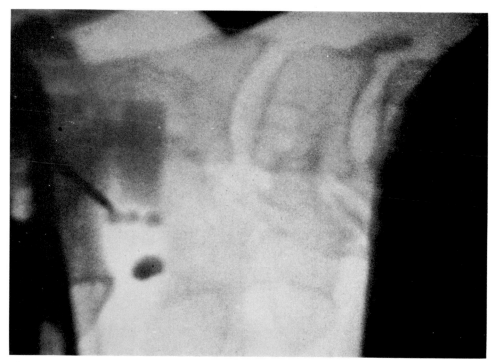

Figure 4-1A. Lateral fluoroscopy showing droplets of Pantopaque resting on dentate ligament, with needle tip immediately adjacent.

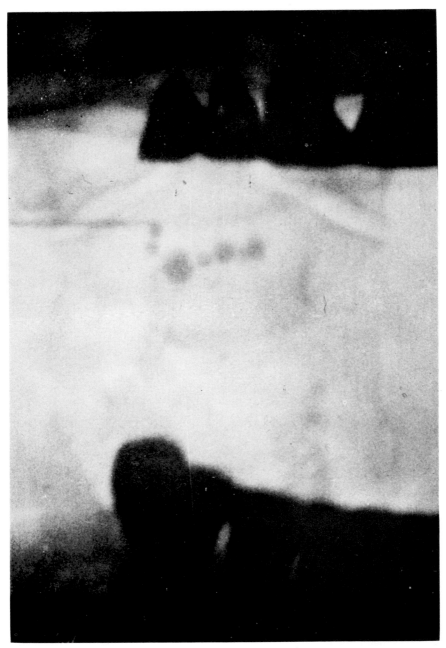

Figure 4-1B. AP fluoroscopy demonstrating tip of needle electrode on dentate ligament just lateral to spinal cord; Pantopaque droplets by needle tip identify lateral margin of cord.

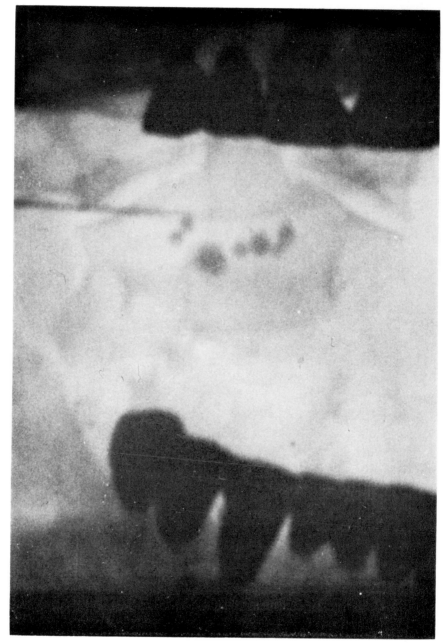

Figure 4-1C. AP fluoroscopy demonstrates displacement of Pantopaque droplet along edge of cord as needle is advanced and cord displaced.

graphic survey, has not given uniformly satisfactory relief of pain following creation of a lesion. Stimulation to verify position in the spinothalmic
tract is the criterion that is used. When appropriate contralateral "tingling" on stimulation is obtained, a satisfactory sensory level is achieved.
The results with percutaneous cordotomy are comparable with those observed after surgical technique (4, 11). The complications of dysesthesia
appear higher than in surgical cordotomies, but seem to be most preva-
lent in those with repeat procedures, as noted by the authors and others
(13).

The role of surgical cordotomy in our practice has changed, but not
disappeared. Percutaneous cordotomy is utilized as a primary procedure.
Surgical cordotomy is carried out if relief is not forthcoming after the
percutaneous method. Bilateral percutaneous cordotomies are carried out
at ten-day intervals in patients with malignancies if the initial sensory
level is not above the nipple line. If a higher level should be obtained or
required, thoracic surgical cordotomy is performed for the second side.
The authors have had no experience with the low cervical anterior approach of Lin (6).

Advantages of the lateral approach are primarily: ready access to cord,
supine position of patient, and no need to traverse areas of cord unrelated
to pain pathways. The problems of cord mobility and rotation, however, may be greater from this approach. Study of the dynamics of cord
deformity and verification of electrode position by evoked potential will,
perhaps, add to the reliability of the procedure.

SUMMARY

The authors' experience and technique with the lateral approach in
121 percutaneous cordotomies upon eighty-three patients is presented.
The results that have been obtained are comparable to those following
surgical cordotomy. The percutaneous method of cordotomy is now the
initial procedure of choice.

REFERENCES

1. BEER, E.: Relief of intractable and persistent pain due to metastases pressing on
nerve plexuses by section of opposite anterolateral column of spinal cord above
entrance of involved nerves. *JAMA*, 60:267, 1913.
2. CRUE, B. L.; TODD, E. M., and CARREGAL, E. J. A.: Posterior approach for high
cervical percutaneous radiofrequency cordotomy. *Confin Neurol*, 30:41, 1968.
3. FRAZIER, C. H.: Section of anterolateral column of spinal cord for relief of pain.
Report of six cases. *Arch Neurol (Chicago)*, 4:137, 1920.
4. GRANT, F. C., and WOOD, F. A.: Experiences with cordotomy. *Clin Neurosurg*, 5:38,
1957.

5. GROFF, R. A.; PITTS, F. W., and MEREDITH, R. C.: Cordotomy: A refinement in technique. *Surg Clin N Amer,* 42:1575, 1962.

6. LIN, P. M.; GILDENBERG, P. L., and POLAKOFF, P. P.: An anterior approach to percutaneous lower cervical cordotomy. *J Neurosurg,* 25:553, 1966.

7. MULLAN, S.; HARPER, P. V.; HEKMATPANAH, J.; TONES, H., and DOBBIN, G.: Percutaneous interruption of spinal-pain tracts by means of a strontium 90 needle. *J Neurosurg,* 20:931, 1963.

8. MULLAN, S.; HEKMATPANAH, J.; DOBBIN, G., and BECKMAN, F.: Percutaneous intramedullary cordotomy utilizing the unipolar anodal electrolytic lesion. *J Neurosurg,* 22:548, 1965.

9. PEET, M. M.: Control of intractable pain in lumbar region, pelvis, and lower extremities by section of anterolateral columns of spinal cord (chordotomy). *Arch Surg (Chicago),* 13:1953, 1926.

10. ROSOMOFF, H. L.; CARROLL, F.; BROWN, J., and SHEPTAK, P.: Percutaneous radiofrequency cervical cardotomy: Technique. *J Neurosurg,* 23:639, 1965.

11. SCHWARTZ, H. G.: High cervical cordotomy—Technique and results. *Clin Neurosurg,* 8:282, 1960.

12. SPILLER, W. G., and MARTIN, E.: The treatment of persistent pain of organic origin in the lower part of the body by division of the anterolateral column of the spinal cord. *JAMA,* 58:1489, 1912.

13. UIHLEIN, A.; WEERASOORIUA, L. A., and HOLMAN, C. B.: Percutaneous electric cervical cordotomy for relief of intractable pain. *Mayo Clin Proc,* 44:176, 1969.

Chapter 5

POSTERIOR APPROACH FOR HIGH CERVICAL PERCUTANEOUS RADIOFREQUENCY STEREOTAXIC CORDOTOMY

BENJAMIN L. CRUE, JR., EDWIN M. TODD, ENRIQUE J. A. CARREGAL, WILLIAM H. WRIGHT AND DAVID B. MALINE

T HE feasibility of percutaneous high cervical cordotomy at the C1-C2 level, utilizing the lateral approach, as introduced by Mullan *et al.* (5) and Rosomoff *et al.* (6, 7), has now been well documented. An anterior approach for percutaneous lower cervical cordotomy for the relief of pain in the trunk or lower extremities has been presented previously

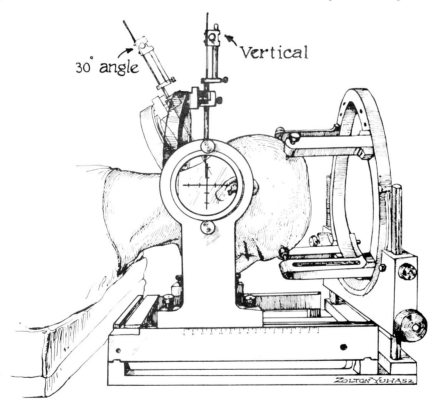

Figure 5-1A. Schematic drawing, lateral view, of the posterior approach (the patient prone in Todd-Wells stereotaxic guide) for trigeminal tractotomy (angled up 30° above the arch of C1) and for posterior cordotomy through the spinal cord (vertical electrode placement between C1-C2).

by Lin *et al.* (4). The present authors have reported (3, 9) that it is also possible to perform a radiofrequency (1, 8) percutaneous cordotomy at the upper cervical level via a posterior approach.

Having previously utilized the posterior approach in the high cervical area for percutaneous trigeminal tractotomy (2), utilization of a similar approach to the anterior quadrant of the spinal cord was contemplated (Fig. 5-1). With the patient in the prone position, a #18 needle was passed straight downwards between the arches of C1 and C2. After spinal fluid was obtained, a #22 coated, sharp-pointed electrode was passed entirely through the spinal cord (certainly a theoretical disadvantage). Having attempted this in the cat in the laboratory prior to utilizing it in the human, it was observed that on some occasions there would be considerable coagulum on the electrode tip when it was withdrawn through the entire depth of the cervical cord. This could be avoided by rotating the electrode prior to its withdrawal.

It was apparent from studies of the human cadaver that the midline of the odontoid usually corresponded well with the midline of the spinal cord if the head and neck were in a neutral position. It was discovered that the cord was usually carried downward and the pia was impinged when the tip of the electrode during slow insertion struck the firm surface of the anterior floor of the canal. This gave a good anterior landmark (Fig. 5-2). The needle was withdrawn 1 to 2 mm and the radiofrequency lesion was started at this point. A line 3.5 mm from the mid-

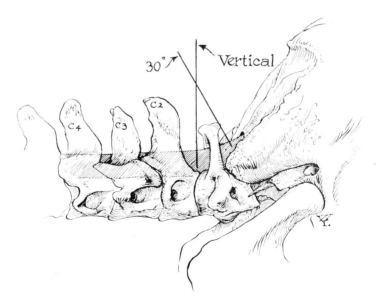

Figure 5-1B. Drawing showing bony detail.

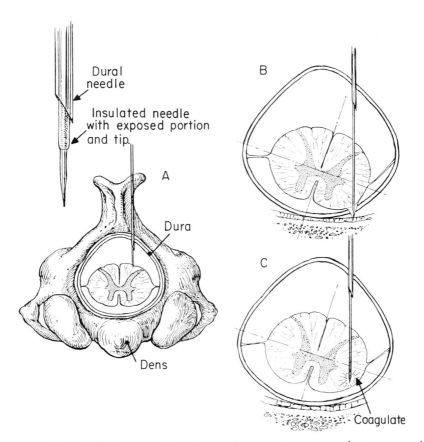

Figure 5-2. Seriographic demonstration of posterior percutaneous cordotomy procedure.

line, as measured in the PA x-ray view, accepting the center of the odontoid as the theoretical center of the cervical cord (Fig. 5-3), was used
as the initial target in the human.

To date, since 1966, the authors have used this posterior approach for
high cervical cordotomy at the C1-C2 level in nineteen patients. This includes bilateral one-stage lesions in two patients, and a unilateral lesion
in seventeen patients. Eighteen patients had verified uncontrolled advanced neoplastic disease. The remaining patient, aged seventy-four, with
long-standing phantom pain in an absent upper extremity, had not responded to conservative measures nor to previous surgical procedures including rhizotomy. He also had an incidental carcinoma of the kidney.
Each of the nineteen patients was placed in a prone position, with the
head held in the Todd-Wells stereotaxic head-holder. They were given
minimal local anesthesia and light sedation.

In two early patients a bilateral procedure was employed at one stage

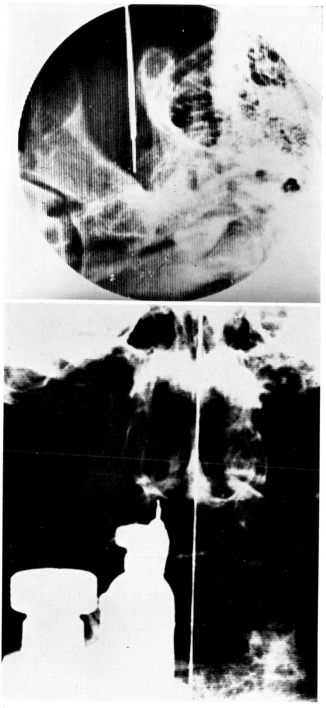

Figure 5-3. Roentgenograph of the #18 needle and electrode inserted in place (in the lateral and AP view) for percutaneous posterior high cervical cordotomy.

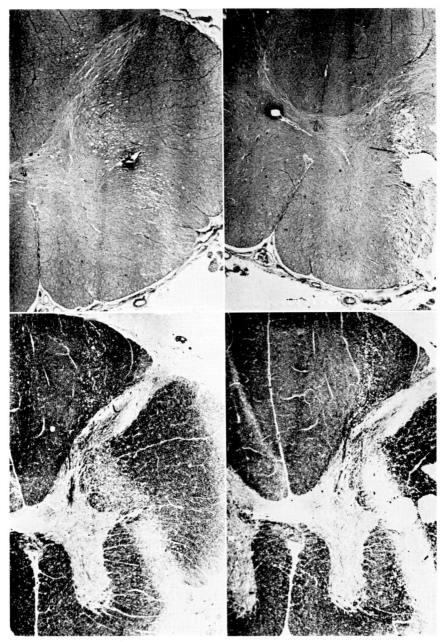

Figure 5-4. Autopsy specimen from the C1-C2 level on patient S. M., undergoing posterior cordotomy. Upper left: Hematoxylin and eosin stain of lesion at the most rostral end of the radiofrequency lesion, showing maximum needle tract in the dorsal column. Upper right: H & E stain at the site of maximum lesion, showing most extensive destruction in the anterior quadrant, with cavitation at or dorsal to the level of the dentate ligament, in the region of the pyramidal tract. Lower left: Loyez myelin stain on paraffin section from the same block as in upper left. Lower right: Same myelin stain at the level of maximum lesion, same block as upper right.

by this posterior approach. In one of these patients a good level of analgesia and subsequent clinical relief of pain was obtained only on one side. The other patient did well for a short time with bilateral pain relief, but on the third postoperative day she lapsed into coma and twenty-four hours later expired quietly. There was no respiratory arrest or nighttime respiratory cessation in either patient. The one mortality was, in all probability, attributable to extensive neoplastic disease; but for the record it must be listed as a postoperative surgical mortality.

There was no mortality and only one serious morbidity in the seventeen patients who had a unilateral C1-C2 posterior percutaneous cordotomy. One patient with carcinoma of the lung invading the brachial plexus had, postoperatively, considerable spastic hemiparesis ipsilateral to the radiofrequency lesion. There was good initial pain relief in all seventeen patients, although it was not total in six. Furthermore, there was the unexpected finding of relief from pain without a dense area of analgesia to pinprick in several cases. This finding has been discussed previously (3). On occasion, the level of sensory loss to pinprick evolved and increased slowly over the first few postoperative days.

The procedure may not give complete relief from pain even in these cancer patients, if the survival from their neoplastic disease has been prolonged. There are three patients who, several months after this type of cordotomy, have once again complained of pain (even though in one of them there was still a good level of dense hypalgesia to pinprick). There were several patients who began to complain postoperatively of pain on the opposite, preoperatively painless or less painful side of the body. To date no patient in this series has undergone a repeat percutaneous cordotomy.

Photographs of a pathological specimen from one patient who survived unilateral posterior cordotomy for seventeen days are shown in Figures 5-4 and 5-5. The absence of any right-sided hemiparesis or even pathological reflex, in view of the demonstrated lesion extending more dorsally than had been intended and in the region of the pyramidal tract, should be mentioned in this particular case. This raises questions about the neuroanatomical and neurophysiological specificity of this region. The need to know more about the physical parameters of radiofrequency lesions in human spinal cord tissue is clearly indicated.

The observation of slowly rising sensory levels after radiofrequency cordotomy has previously been noted. While, perhaps, more understandable in lesions produced with strontium 90, the pathogenesis is more difficult to envision when radiofrequency current is used. The finding of clinical relief of pain without good sensory level or even, in a few cases,

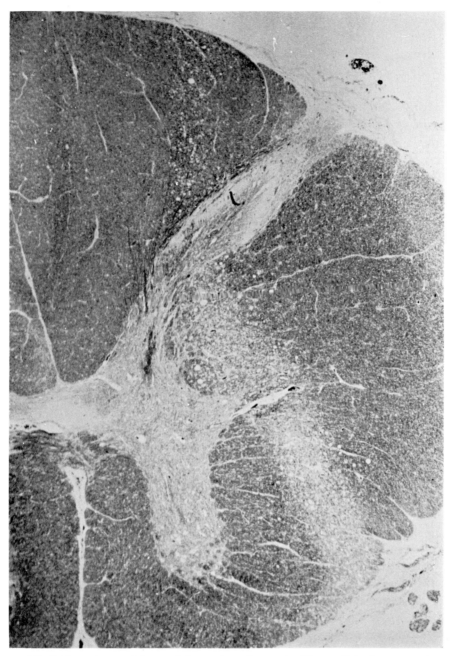

Figure 5-5. Enlargement of lower left section shown in Figure 5-4, demonstrating the maximum damage in the dorsal column from passage of the #22 needle electrode, in and out.

much sensory loss to pinprick test deserves some comment. Further attempts to obtain a better classical sensory level have been continued by the surgeon when only a poor level is noted during percutaneous cordotomy under local anesthesia. This is usually done in the belief that anything short of the expected result will not be satisfactory because there may be only short-term clinical benefit. Since the cases reported in this paper are still too few in number, and all but one were done in patients with terminal malignancy, a comment on long-term results in patients without good sensory level cannot be made. In several of the patients with less than satisfactory sensory levels postcordotomy, however, there has been relief from pain until demise. This raises questions about the mechanisms that are involved in such responses. It is possible that any significant quantitative decrease in afferent inflow cephalad in the appropriate cord area may give relief to some degree, with length of time for the satisfactory result a variable that is yet to be determined. This could be thought of as analogous to the compression procedure on the trigeminal posterior root in tic douloureux. It suggests at least further refinement of the cordotomy technique to take into account the individual patients, many of whom may be victims of far-advanced neoplasms.

In three of the most recent unilateral posterior cordotomies that were done for patients with bronchogenic carcinoma involving the brachial plexus, the authors were able, by going slightly more medially (2.0 to 3.0 mm from midline), to effect good relief from pain with sensory loss to pin only in the arm and shoulder, sparing the lower trunk and lower extremity. It has been more difficult to extend laterally, i.e. to get the lower extremity as numb as the upper extremity and shoulder, without sliding off the cord in the attempt. It is possible that the posterior approach through the cord and into the medial anterior quadrant may be appropriate in the treatment of patients with carcinoma involving the brachial plexus or upper extremity, whereas a lateral approach may remain superior for obtaining pain relief in the lower trunk and lower extremity. The postmortem specimens examined to date have shown that it is quite feasible to pass the needle electrode through the dorsal columns with minimal damage to the cord. The electrode used in these studies is a #22 needle size having a .025 inch diameter. With an exposed 2 mm tip, this gives a good radiofrequency lesion in the anterior quadrant, usually at 100 milliamps for about twenty to thirty seconds (Radionics, Mode A).

Whether the posterior approach for percutaneous stereotaxic cordotomy will prove to be safe and whether it will have any real advantage over the lateral approach must await the accumulation of further data. At present the authors are convinced that their technique of unilateral high cervical cordotomy is worthy of continuation, especially for treating patients with previously vexatious bronchogenic carcinomas invading the brachial plexus and shoulder region.

The authors have also been interested in attempting to obtain reliable neurophysiological data from this high cervical cord, utilizing the electrode for recording prior to making the radiofrequency destructive lesion. It is believed that this posterior approach affords a unique opportunity to monitor impulses both in the dorsal posterior columns in the human cord and then ventrally in the anterior quadrant. Attempts are being made to record responses while both intensifying the patient's pain and while using physiological pain and touch stimuli below the cervical area, as well as during electrical stimulation in the lower extremities. So far the results have added very little to our knowledge, and technically leave much to be desired. At present the data are being recorded on magnetic tape and fed into a computer of averaged transients in an attempt to obtain more meaningful records from these patients suffering from carcinomatous disease.

REFERENCES

1. BRODKEY, J. S.; MIYAZAKI, Y.; ERVIN, F. R., and MARK, V. H.: Reversible heat lesions with radiofrequency current. *J Neurosurg*, 21:49, 1964.
2. CRUE, B. L.; TODD, E. M.; CARREGAL, E. J. A., and KILHAM, O.: Percutaneous trigeminal tractotomy—Case report utilizing stereotactic radiofrequency lesion. *Bull Los Angeles Neurol Soc*, 32:86, 1967.
3. CRUE, B. L.; TODD, E. M., and CARREGAL, E. J. A.: Posterior approach for high cervical percutaneous radiofrequency cordotomy. *Confin Neurol*, 30:41, 1968.
4. LIN, P. M.; GILDENBERG, P. L., and POLAKOFF, P. P.: An anterior approach to percutaneous lower cervical cordotomy. *J Neurosurg*, 25:553, 1966.
5. MULLAN, S.; HARPER, P. V.; HEKMATPANAH, J.; TORRES, H., and DOBBIN, G.: Percutaneous interruption of spinal pain-tracts by means of a strontium-90 needle. *J Neurosurg*, 20:931, 1963.
6. ROSOMOFF, H. L.; CARROLL, F.; BROWN, J., and SHEPTAK, P.: Percutaneous radiofrequency cervical cordotomy: Technique. *J Neurosurg*, 23:639, 1965.
7. ROSOMOFF, H. L.; SHEPTAK, P., and CARROLL, F.: Modern pain relief: Percutaneous chordotomy. *JAMA*, 196:482, 1966.
8. SWEET, W. H.; MARK, V. H., and HAMLIN, H.: Radiofrequency lesions in the central nervous system of man and cat. *J Neurosurg*, 17:213, 1960.
9. TODD, E. M.; CRUE, B. L., and CARREGAL, E. J. A.: Posterior percutaneous tractotomy and cordotomy. *Confin Neurol* (in press).

Chapter 6

MICROSURGICAL RHIZOTOMY IN
TRIGEMINAL NEURALGIA

PETER J. JANNETTA*

PEOPLE come to a physician because they want to feel better. Pain is a common presenting symptom from which the patient wants relief. The pain of trigeminal neuralgia has been, in general, best relieved by retrogasserian rhizotomy as perfected by the Spiller-Frazier (8, 9) technique which results in the lowest recurrence rate of pain of any procedure and a low morbidity rate. However, postoperative numbness can be as disabling to the patient as the pain was previously—autonomic dysfunction in the skin, although rare, is a dread problem; first division pain is not adequately treated without the threat of complications in the eye.

Retrogasserian rhizotomy performed through the posterior fossa has been successful for many years, but with a slightly higher mortality rate than the middle fossa approach to the nerve. Preservation of sensation, especially light touch sensation, has been a variably present bonus with this technique. A strong hint as to etiology of the symptoms of trigeminal neuralgia has been presented by Dandy (3-5), who found a high incidence of vascular abnormalities about the trigeminal nerve at the pons, using gross techniques without magnification through the posterior fossa route.

The transtentorial microsurgical approach appears to be useful in certain cases (6). It permits selective section of the portio major, with visualization and safe preservation of the motor rootlets and the associated sensory fascicles ("accessory fibers" of Dandy [3-5], "intermediate fibers") that appear to carry so much light touch and corneal sensation, while producing hypalgesia and pain relief. It is especially valuable in first division trigeminal neuralgia, as the corneal reflex and sensation may be normal or only slightly diminished after a total portio major transsection at the pons. The technique permits visualization of what is possibly the primary etiology in trigeminal neuralgia: compression-distortion of the trigeminal nerve at the pons, usually by vascular structures such as tortuous branches of the superior cerebellar artery or by tumor. The morbidity appears low in a small series of patients. The consequences of temporal

* Supported in part by NIH Grant 1-R01-NBO 7095-NEUA.

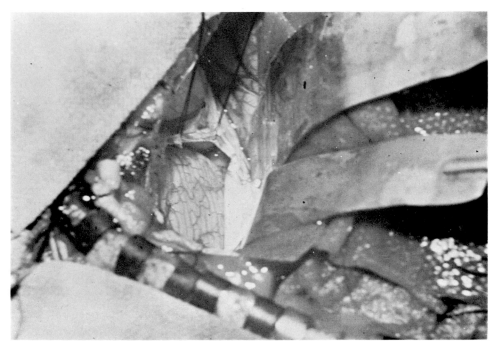

Figure 6-1. View of a left temporal cranial area prepared for exploration of trigeminal nerve and upper cerebellopontine angle. Pictured is an extensive exposure used for a patient with a tumor in the region. The temporal lobe was elevated over Telfa-covered cottonoids using self-retaining retractors. A wide opening in the tentorium is seen with the petrous ridge just above two stay-sutures in the tentorium. The anteromedial superior surface of the cerebellum is seen through the opening in the tentorium, with the trigeminal nerve seen just superomedial to this. Much less elevation of the temporal lobe and retraction is necessary in trigeminal neuralgia which can be done with one retractor, modest temporal lobe elevation and preservation of most bridging veins.

lobe elevation, especially if many bridging veins to the lateral sinus are taken or if the vein of Labbe (which should be preserved) is sacrificed, should be the only major source of postoperative morbidity.

The technique (6) consists of a temporal craniotomy with the patient in the lateral position and premedicated with adrenal steroids. The patient is given an osmotic diuretic. A free bone flap is turned, the dura mater is opened and anterior bridging veins are coagulated and divided as necessary for elevation of the temporal lobe over the petrous ridge into the area of the anterior tentorium cerebelli. A self-retaining retractor is put into place after the incisura of the tentorium is inspected. High retraction of the temporal lobe is not necessary. It is important that Telfa-covered cottonoids or a rubber dam be placed against the temporal lobe for retraction so that brain tissue and bridging posterior temporal veins are not torn. Still using gross dissection and with the self-retaining retractor in place, an incision is made behind the petrous ridge about half the distance between the incisura and the lateral sinus. Care must be taken to stay behind the superior petrosal sinus (Fig. 6-1). Multiple incisions are made in a triangular fashion to dissect anteromedially, and when the free edge of the antero medial cerebellum is reached the microscope is brought into play. A small bridging vein is usually found in this region extending from the anteromedial superior aspect of the cerebellum to the superior petrosal sinus just lateral to the trigeminal nerve. The cerebellum may need to be retracted minimally, but this has not usually been the case. The trigeminal nerve is seen entering and leaving the dural canal and the pons quite high and anterior in the posterior fossa. Any abnormalities about the nerve may be easily identified (Fig. 6-2), using 10X or 16X magnification. Inferolateral section of the portio major is then carried out, 70 to 100 percent of the cross-sectional area of the portio major being taken with preservation of all other fascicles. In several instances the author has been able to move vessels away from the trigeminal nerve and, in one patient, this alone was done as the treatment of choice. The tentorial defect is left open, the retractor and cottonoids are removed and the wound is closed in the usual fashion without drainage. Postoperative care is as with any routine craniotomy.

Sixteen patients with classical trigeminal neuralgia intractable to good medical therapy have been operated upon using the above technique. They ranged in age from twenty-eight to seventy-three years. Definite compression-distortion of the trigeminal nerve at the pons was present in fifteen of the sixteen patients. Vascular compression-distortion was found in twelve of the patients, usually due to tortuous elongated branches of the superior cerebellar artery that appeared to have been caught in pia arachnoid in such a way as to slide down the belly of the pons from above and so impinge on the trigeminal nerve at the site of its entry and exit from the midportion of the pons. One patient was found to have a small pontine glioma that invaded the trigeminal nerve roots. Another was found to have a meningioma of the cerebellopontine angle arising from the medial petrous ridge and compressing and distorting the trigeminal nerve. Another was found to have a large arteriovenous malformation compressing and distorting the trigeminal nerve in the same region. The sixteenth patient had numerous tortuous arteries around the trigeminal nerve at the pons, but no compression-distortion could be seen. The trigeminal nerve was small and atrophic, probably secondary to a previous middle fossa operation.

The pain recurred in the patient with the pontine glioma whose tumor

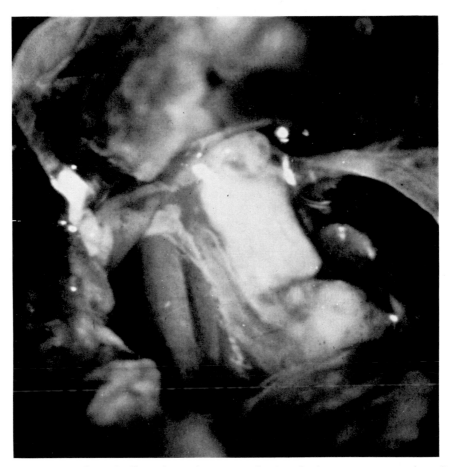

Figure 6-2. View through dissecting microscope of trigeminal nerve at operation. Pons and cerebellum are below, trigeminal nerve enters dural canal in center above median point of photograph. From left to right are seen the elevated temporal lobe, the opening in the tentorium, two vascular loops that were compressing and distorting the trigeminal nerve at pons, motor and intermediate branches of trigeminal nerve, portio major of trigeminal nerve with transverse incision through its entirety, and another vascular loop to the right of the nerve.

was very vascular. Excessive bleeding was frightening when the nerve was sectioned, and, therefore, a probably inadequate section was performed. A standard Spiller-Frazier trigeminal nerve section has subsequently been done with resultant relief of pain. First division pain developed in the patient with the arteriovenous malformation of the posterior fossa, whose previous pain had been located in the region of the third division. A partial portio major transsection had been performed in this patient a bit further out on the root than is usually done because the malformation was so extensive around the trigeminal nerve at the pons. There have been no other recurrences of the pain of trigeminal neuralgia to date in a follow-up of three to thirty-nine months.

The mechanism of pain in trigeminal neuralgia is poorly understood. There may be a biphasic arrangement in that mechanical compression-distortion of the nerve may be the first event and may trigger the changes of hypermyelination and hypomyelination seen on electron microscopy by Beaver, *et al.* (1, 2), and Kerr and Miller (7).

Our preliminary experience with the relief of trigeminal neuralgia using the transtentorial microsurgical approach to the nerve at the pons would appear to contribute information about this mechanism. Of great interest is one patient in whom the tortuous artery was mobilized away from the trigeminal nerve without touching the nerve at any time. The patient awoke without pain only to suffer a recurrence three months after her operation, with onset at the time she was thrown from a horse. The patient was treated with Dilantin with excellent results and she has remained free of pain with no medication for over two years.

REFERENCES

1. BEAVER, D. L.; MOSES, H. L., and GANOT, C. E.: Electron microscopy of the trigeminal ganglion. II Autopsy study of human ganglia. *Arch Path (Chicago)*, 79:557, 1965.
2. BEAVER, D. L.; MOSES, H. L., and GANOTE, C. E.: Electron microscopy of the trigeminal ganglion. III Trigeminal neuralgia. *Arch Path (Chicago)*, 79:571, 1965.
3. DANDY, W. E.: The treatment of trigeminal neuralgia by the cerebellar route. *Ann Surg*, 96:787, 1932.
4. DANDY, W. E.: Concerning the cause of trigeminal neuralgia. *Amer J Surg*, 24:447, 1934.
5. DANDY, W. E.: Trigeminal neuralgia and trigeminal tic douloureux. In: Lewis, D. (Ed.): *Practice of Surgery*. Hagerstown, Md., Prior, 1963, vol. 12, pp. 167-187.
6. JANNETTA, P. J., and RAND, R. W.: Transtentorial retrogasserian rhizotomy in trigeminal neuralgia by microsurgical technique. *Bull Los Angeles Neurol Soc*, 31:93, 1966.
7. KERR, F. W. L., and MILLER, R. H.: The pathology of trigeminal neuralgia. Electron microscope studies. *Arch Neurol (Chicago)*, 15:308, 1966.
8. SPILLER, W. G., and Frazier, C. H.: The division of sensory root of the trigeminus for relief of tic douloureux; an experimental, pathological and clinical study with a preliminary report of one surgically successful case. *Philadelphia Med J*, 8:1039, 1901.
9. SPILLER, W. G., and FRAZIER, C. H.: Tic douloureux: Anatomic and clinical basis for subtotal section of sensory root of trigeminal nerve. *Arch Neurol (Chicago)*, 29:50, 1933.

Chapter 7

OBSERVATIONS ON THE PRESENT STATUS OF THE COMPRESSION PROCEDURE IN TRIGEMINAL NEURALGIA

Benjamin L. Crue, Jr., Edwin M. Todd and Enrique J. A. Carregal

THE treatment of patients who have primary trigeminal neuralgia (tic douloureux) has finally entered that long sought phase of effective medical therapy with the realization that several of the anticonvulsant medications do, indeed, have a beneficial therapeutic effect in this painful condition (8, 24). As Penman (47) has recently pointed out, Peter, in 1876, treated tic douloureux with potassium bromide. The present senior author (13), as early as 1954 prescribed Dilantin (sodium diphenyl hydantoin) for patients with tic pain, based on the hypothesis that it appeared on clinical grounds alone that trigeminal neuralgia was, as often mentioned by earlier medical writers, a true form of epilepsy (12). Instead of being a motor disorder it appeared to involve the sensory system, presumably in the region of the central trigeminal nuclear complex in the lower brain stem. In usual clinical doses Dilantin did not appear to be efficacious, and this medical attempt was abandoned. However, others (28) (although they prescribed it for different reasons) were more perspicacious and tenacious and did demonstrate that there was clinical improvement in certain patients with tic douloureux who were given Dilantin. The medical armamentarium was further improved by King's (33) suggestion of adding Tolseram (5) (mephenesin carbamate). His later follow-up (34), as well as one by the present authors (20), verified that Dilantin and Tolseram could hold the pain reasonably in check and obviate the need for surgical intervention in approximately two-thirds of the patients with tic douloureux. More recently, Bloom (4) has added Tegretol (carbamazepine) to the armamentarium. At the present time, it would appear that in spite of the controversy that still exists concerning the etiology of tic douloureux, this condition in most cases responds clinically to medical management.

There remains for surgical consideration a definite group of patients with true tic pain who either are not controlled by present pharmaceutical means or who have developed an allergy to the medications utilized. This minority, at the present time, still has to be approached from the same previous viewpoint—exactly what type of operation (71)

47

is best suited for each patient? The authors of this paper utilize initial alcohol block, especially in 2nd division tic pain and the rarer 1st division pain, for patients in whom superficial infraorbital or supraorbital nerve injection often gives adequate, though usually temporary, relief. The deep 2nd or 3rd division block is no longer used except in very elderly patients or those who are poor risks. If the patient's condition is satisfactory with present-day general anesthesia, surgical intervention is usually recommended quite promptly. It is in this group of patients that the trigeminal compression procedure would seem to have still a definite role.

Following a suggestion made by Woltman *et al.* (72), a search was begun by Shelden *et al.* (53) for a means of alleviating tic pain surgically, without the postoperative annoying facial anesthesia. An intracranial decompression of the trigeminal nerve was carried out at the foramen rotundum or foramen ovale by means of a dental drill in patients with tic pain in the 2nd or 3rd division. A series of ten cases was done, with good relief of pain in all cases; but, there was a prompt recurrence in the majority. The technique of Taarnhoj (26, 64) in decompressing the posterior root had also given excellent results in relieving patients of pain. It appeared that the common denominator between the two decompression procedures might have been trauma to the trigeminal peripheral system sufficient to abolish the pain, but not sufficient enough to result in significant postoperative facial sensory loss. Therefore, a deliberate compression procedure was carried out. For theoretical reasons, in an attempt to make it more permanent, the trauma was directed to the region of the ganglion and posterior root through the standard middle fossa approach (Fig. 7-1).

To date, well over three hundred craniotomies for this compression procedure have been carried out in patients with tic douloureux by Shelden, Pudenz, Freshwater, Crue or Todd. There is no longer any question but that the procedure is effective. There has been surprisingly uniform relief of patients with the clinical tic pain. The main drawback has been a gradually increasing recurrence rate with the passage of time, as had been originally predicted. In 1960, after the first 115 cases, a review revealed approximately a 20 percent pain rate of recurrence (51). While the present recurrence rate is not known precisely it is undoubtedly higher than this, but has remained within acceptable limits because of two factors. First, it would appear that the majority of those patients who are going to have a recurrence of pain seem to have it in the first few years after surgery. Secondly, the recurrence of pain is not quite as upsetting to the patient, or at least to the surgeon, as it was previously. Several of the patients with a recurrence of pain after the compression procedure have been controlled with Dilantin or Tolseram, which had been ineffective prior to the compression procedure.

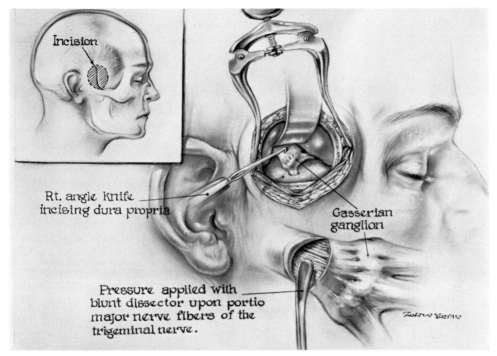

Figure 7-1. Operative exposure and methods of compression of the posterior root fibers (53).

The authors no longer expose the region of the ganglion on the floor of the middle fossa after the extradural approach as widely as was originally illustrated. In recent cases the middle meningeal artery has not been sacrificed routinely, and the region of the ganglion is compressed with a flat metal dissector against the floor of the skull without opening Meckel's cave or inspecting the trigeminal fibers directly. Trigeminal compression remains the standard operative procedure for those patients who are uncontrolled by medical regimen or superficial alcohol block. There are two exceptions. In very elderly patients or in patients with other medical conditions making them poor surgical risks—e.g., cardiac abnormalities, diabetes or other serious concurrent disease—subtotal rhizotomy is employed, with care being taken to cut all of the fibers of the 2nd or 3rd division, sparing only the ophthalmic division. This is done in an attempt to avoid any further surgical procedure from a possible recurrence. If there is significant 1st division pain, then the entire root is sectioned through the middle fossa approach. It has been the writers' experience that these elderly or sick patients are usually troubled very little by the facial or corneal anesthesia, as are the more active younger patients with tic. (Like all generalizations, this is not uniformly true.) The second exception is the occurrence of true tic pain in patients with known multiple sclerosis. In the few cases that have been encountered, this appears to be a different disease. Many of these patients require more extensive operative procedures, and the compression procedure is no longer used even in young patients with disseminated sclerosis.

Further efforts to find a more physiological and nonoperative approach in treating patients with trigeminal neuralgia will be continued by neurosurgeons until a more universally effective and safe pharmaceutical treatment is forthcoming. Percutaneous trigeminal tractotomy (18) will be discussed elsewhere, but this is still a major operation, still experimental, and may well prove to be either too hazardous or ineffective.

Attempts to find a satisfactory nonoperative treatment in patients suffering from chronic pain have led to some interesting approaches. Attempts to further alter the trigeminal system by such techniques as injection of toxins or isotopes into the peripheral trigeminal branches was contemplated by the authors but so far has proven to be impracticable. Recently, added impetus has been supplied by continuing study of the neurophysiology of pain by such investigators as Casey and Melzak (7), Melzak and Wall (42), and Sweet (62). The observation that cutaneous physiological stimuli have an effect on subsequent sensory perception in the human being has been known for a long time. Cold or wind has often been referred to in the literature over the years as a possible etiological factor in the development of Bell's motor palsy. This, of course, still remains unproven, but is certainly an interesting speculation. The observation that such things as wind on the face can affect sensory perception has been less discussed. One of the authors had experienced prolonged hypalgesia to pinprick after driving with an open window and wind blowing on his face. It was thus decided to see whether repetitive electrical stimulation could be used to more permanently influence the sensory system. Cats were utilized during 1958 and 1959 for acute experiments only. No chronic implantations were done. Repetitive stimulation of the peripheral trigeminal system was given over many hours in an attempt to accomplish transneuronal degeneration centrally. These attempts were unsuccessful and never reported.

In 1960 and 1961, utilizing a small mercury eight-volt battery, repetitive stimuli were applied after the same electrode had been used to locate the peripheral cutaneous nerves in patients with neuralgia and phantom limb. The effect produced seemed minimal, short-lived and of no clinical benefit. Electrical stimulation was discarded because it appeared that physiological stimuli were probably more effective. The best clinical success was encountered not in patients with trigeminal neuralgia, but in those with postherpetic neuralgia. It was found that while the jabbing, sudden, sharp tic-like neuralgic pains of postherpetic neuralgia could be controlled by Dilantin in many cases (as could tabetic pains and certain of the cases of phantom limb pain), the more constant dysesthesias, including "burning" pain, appeared resistant to almost all forms of therapy in postherpetic neuralgia. It was found that considerable relief could be obtained by such simple conservative measures as the hand vibrator, ethyl chloride spray or the application of ice cubes over the skin in the region of the postherpetic burning dysesthesia (65) if the patient was psychologically able to have insight into the situation and was treated with tranquilizers or sedation (and, more recently, with the use of antidepressants such as Elavil). It was the authors' impression that they were probably decreasing the afferent input into crucial neurophysiologically active abnormal central connections by activating "overlapping" or "competing" circuits by stimulating the predominantly larger touch fibers, without evoking pain as was done by the old mustard plaster treatment or acupuncture. Recently, a better explanation has been advanced by the much more sophisticated experiments of Wall and Sweet (70). They proposed that stimulation of the larger nonpainful touch fibers, which they successfully carried out electrically, is efficacious by "closing the gate" (42, 43).

Further discussion of the physiology of pain (1, 55, 73) (as well as the possible etiology and pathophysiology in trigeminal neuralgia [61]) is necessary, since understanding of the mechanisms involved would appear to be a prerequisite to advancements in therapy. (Although the two usually go hand in hand; and, quite often, an understanding of the physiology follows serendipitously from involvement in treatment.) Therefore, the authors would like to comment on Melzak and Wall's concept, as it possibly relates to this problem. There may yet be some objections to the gate theory of modulation of pain (40) at the spinal cord level, as evidenced by some recent neurophysiological experiments by Zimmerman (74), and Franz and Iggo (23). Furthermore, this concept, even for "normal" physiological pain, is overly simplified. The possibility of more peripheral modulation by antidromic activity has not been included. This antidromic activity in the form of a dorsal root reflex (67) would appear to be physiological and quantitatively rather important, in the trigeminal system especially (6, 11). Whether it is induced in the primary afferent endings (21, 54, 69) transsynaptically (27) by presynaptic inhibition (22) carried to the extreme (where threshold for firing is reached) still remains to be proven. However, on hypothetical grounds alone this gate theory would also appear to be inadequate, as it does not take into account the prolonged temporal factor observed in certain pathological pain conditions such as neuralgia. It would appear that there must be a postsynaptic central mechanism, regardless of any possible peripheral etiology (2, 25, 32). The prolonged nature of the discharges necessarily underlying continued pain must require repetitive firing of central neurons (35, 39) rather than continuous peripheral "irritation" (30) with bombardment of the central nervous system. Whether this central repetitive discharge is located at a low level in the trigeminal nuclear complex in the case of trigeminal neuralgia, and in the dorsal horn in the region of the substantia gelatinosa in postherpetic neuralgias and other chronic pains of the trunk and extremities, has yet to be proven. Whether the terms "repetitive discharge" (68), "flare," "uncontrolled activity," reverberating circuit, pain "memory" or "engram," feedback or other analogous pseudonyms are used, it can also be considered as epileptiform discharge and is then a type of "sensory epilepsy" (19). The finding of posttetanic potentiation in this sensory system must also be assigned a role (9, 10, 13, 17).

Such "low level" epileptiform activity in the human would seem on clinical grounds to be involved as a basic neurophysiological mechanism in

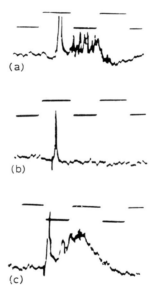

(a)

(b)

(c)

Figure 7-2. Sweep a. Maxillary nerve response at foramen rotundum following 0.6 volt stimulation of infraorbital nerve. Sweep b. When the posterior root of the trigeminal nerve is compressed gently with a cotton pledget the played response is no longer seen while the afferent spike remains. Sweep c. A 30 min. wait followed by an increased stimulus to 15 volts did not bring back the late potential. However, in the posterior root on the proximal side of the compression, the afferent spike was always present. Increasing the stimulus to 4 volts elicited the delayed wave again (13).

many conditions; hiccoughing, torticollis, and ejaculation on the motor side; and on the sensory side would include such syndromes as many forms of vertigo and dizziness, tinnitus, migraine headaches, Horton's cluster headaches, Sluder's lower half sphenopalatine neuralgia, the Barre-Liou syndrome, "parasympathetic storm," sympathetic "irritation," reflex sympathetic dystrophy with Sudex's atrophy, neurogenic leg night cramps, causalgia, "post-traumatic headache" and many different types of neuralgias including postherpetic, tabetic, meralgia paraesthetica and a host of other clinical syndromes.

The authors have on clinical grounds alone long considered the paroxysms of pain in trigeminal neuralgia as a form of sensory epilepsy (12). In an attempt to study the trigeminal central connections neurophysiologically, the delayed antidromic dorsal root potential as described by King *et al.* (36-38), Mamo and Loget (41) and Stewart and his associates (58, 59) has been utilized in a number of experiments—both in cats (Fig. 7-2) and human beings. During 1960 and 1961 some thirty conscious patients with chronic pain had neurophysiological recordings taken from their peripheral trigeminal systems. The most significant finding was the fact that in tic douloureux there was spontaneous activity in the peripheral trigeminal nerves synchronous with the occurrence of subjective tic pain (10). This activity was presumed to be antidromic, and an epiphenomenon mirroring the abnormal central activity that was believed to be a type of epileptiform discharge (Fig. 7-3). Such activity has been demonstrated on the oscilloscope in five of the fourteen tic patients in which peripheral monitoring was attempted.

It is believed that most forms of therapy for patients with neuralgia (15, 17) result in a deactivation centrally (or a "deafferentiation") by quantitatively decreasing arriving afferent potentials from the periphery. Thus triggered or spontaneous uncontrolled firing in this central epileptiform focus no longer occurs. This is a confusing concept, since originally "deafferentiation" (or alteration of the peripheral afferent sensory input code) probably played an important etiological role in establishment of the neurophysiologically active central abnormal focus. How repetitive or reverberating circuits in the region of the trigeminal central complex (31) would differ from those in the cord in the region of substantia gelatinosa (48, 63) remains to be explained. Why peripheral physiological touch stimulation would appear to work clinically in certain cases of postherpetic neuralgia, either by activating competing circuits or by closing the gate, and yet trigger pain in patients with trigeminal neuralgia also remains unexplained. Why tic patients often press (sometimes with masochistic glee) on the area where they had shortly before experienced

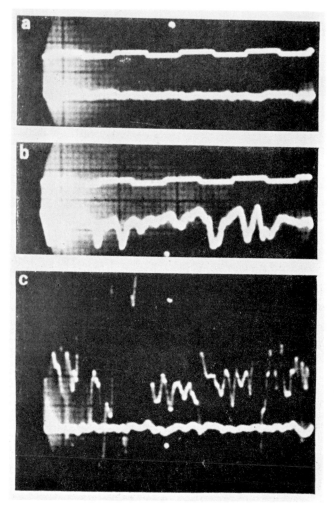

Figure 7-3. a. Monopolar recording from the infraorbital nerve in relaxed human patient. No stimulus. 8 msec time line. b. Same as above only spontaneous tic pain in left second division. c. Bottom line as in above recordings. Upper beam recording electromyographic potentials from left facial muscles during active voluntary contraction. Amplitude sensitivity unchanged in all three bottom sweeps (10).

a severe jabbing pain is puzzling, especially since prior to the sensation they were afraid to touch even lightly that area for fear of triggering a paroxysm of pain (14).

Further elucidation of electrical parameters in attempts to obtain further knowledge about the alleviation of pain are, perhaps, going to open up a whole new avenue of approach. Reports concerning electrical stimulation from workers such as Sweet and Wall are awaited eagerly. Electrical

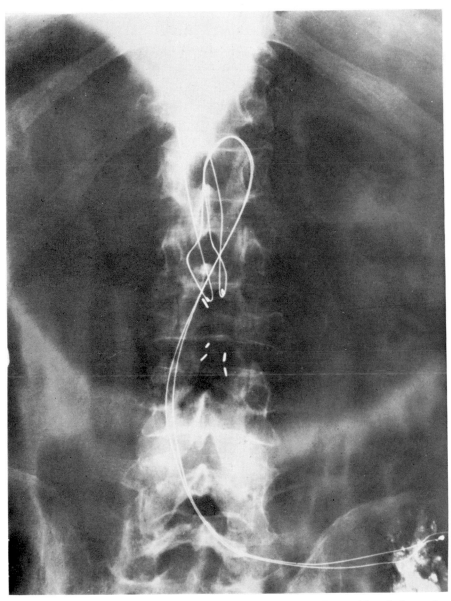

Figure 7-4. AP x-ray view of City of Hope patient demonstrating epidural electrodes for "electrical cordotomy" by repetitive "blocking" stimuli placed at the time of open laminectomy done for decompression of block from collapse of the L3 vertebra from metastatic carcinoma primary in the kidney.

nerve-blocking devices as described by Shelden, Pudenz and Doyle (52) will certainly undergo further utilization. The possibility of operation for implantation of repetitive stimulating electrodes acting directly upon the dorsal cord has been reported by Shealy *et al.* (49, 50) and is certainly an important contribution. In an attempt to utilize (and test) Shealy's observations, it was decided to pass cephalad epidural insulated wire electrodes in patients undergoing decompressive laminectomy for metastatic spinal cord compression. This would obviate the need for a separate open surgical approach. Figure 7-4 reveals such an attempt with the electrodes placed posteriorly (but not quite symmetrically) in the epidural space at the cauda level. In this patient they were left in place for ten days and then pulled out without complication. Until we are certain of the advantages of electrical stimulation as a form of cordotomy, we do not plan to utilize buried subcutaneous induction coils. In this particular patient postoperative testing was most limited, but there did seem to be pain relief. A square wave of 2 to 3 volts scale, .2 msec duration and at a rate of 100 stimuli per second appeared to be effective in this case. It is to be hoped that physical parameters, perhaps, can be elucidated in the future that will work by stimulating at the skin surface, circumventing the need for any type of surgical intervention. This is at present the goal of the authors' neurophysiological inquiry into pain mechanisms. At least implantation of electrodes for pain control may be done stereotaxically (44-46, 66); and, in the cord in the cervical region, percutaneously (16). Figure 7-5 demonstrates the placement of bilateral epidural electrodes by percutaneous stereotaxic technique, similar to the procedure used in cordotomy at the C1-2 level with the patient prone in the Todd-Wells headrest under sedation and local anesthesia only, utilizing the posterior approach. In this case the parameters used for electrical stimulation were the square wave at 100 per sec, .3 msec duration, from 3 to 8 volts scale. Higher voltage was well tolerated but did not appear as effective. The patient appeared to have decreased sensation to pinprick below this level when the current was on, although she could not subjectively tell when it was on or off. She was rapidly weaned from MS gr 1/4 q 2 hrs and was on no pain medications for the sixteen days the electrodes were left in place.

The anatomy of the trigeminal system (56, 57), as well as the physiology (60), requires further detailed investigation. An interesting approach to the posterior trigeminal root, using the operating microscope, has been advocated recently by Jannetta and Rand (29). This is certainly an intriguing surgical approach and an interesting use of the binocular microscope. While their results appear satisfactory, Jannetta and Rand's

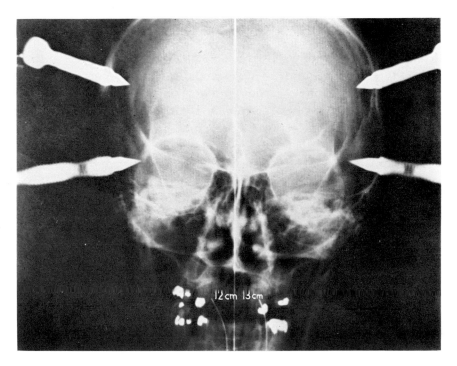

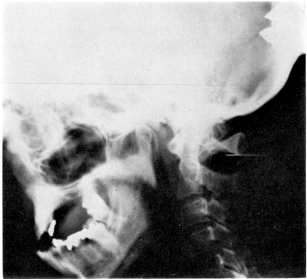

Figure 7-5. AP and lateral x-ray views of bilateral epidural electrodes in another City of Hope patient with lower extremity pain from metastatic carcinoma of the cervix. These electrodes were placed at the Cl-2 level stereotaxically and percutaneously.

interpolation of the functional anatomy, based on the presumed physiology as interpreted from their clinical findings following sparing of the trigeminal accessory roots, is not acceptable at this time. There are, in a number of individuals, accessory rootlets between the pars major and the motor pars minor in the trigeminal root as described by Dandy. There is as yet no anatomical or experimental physiological evidence to show that they have any modality-specific function. While it is to be expected, perhaps, that some of the rootlets running with the pars minor may be sensory from the mesencephalic tract and may carry proprioception from the muscles of mastication, it is not believed that the other accessory roots have any disproportionate number of large touch fibers, leaving the pain fibers in the pars major. The authors with Sutin and Cravioto (unpublished data) have made a study of the root entry zone and central connections in cats, rats and human beings (including three patients previously operated upon for trigeminal neuralgia), utilizing both myelin degeneration and Nauta stains. They were unable to demonstrate any specific division of fibers. Therefore, until further evidence is obtained with better anatomical demonstration in this region it would appear that Jannetta's results in tic patients, like Dandy's partial root section, may be due merely to a quantitative decrease in the summating (3) afferent input to the postulated epileptic central focus. This would explain Jannetta's clinical results, which are similar to those seen following the compression procedure, i.e., tic pain is abolished, but there is preservation to touch and often a relative hypalgesia to pinprick in the face. If this hypothesis is true it should be possible to do the opposite of Jannetta's procedure, by cutting the accessory roots (where they are found to be large) and leaving the sensory pars major. It would be anticipated that identical postoperative facial sensory findings would be demonstrated, and if there were enough fibers in the accessory rootlets that had been cut, the tic pain should also be abolished. This should prove an interesting experiment.*

To summarize our present concept, even "normal" pain cannot be considered as a specific primary sensory modality. There must be some type of central mechanism, both presynaptic and post synaptic, for modulation and final integration of summating inputs from varied peripheral adequate stimuli. Specificity and pattern theory have yet to be satisfactorily combined. Chronic "abnormal" pain states, especially in non-malignant conditions, present a very complex problem with many clinically recognized modulating parameters, both inhibiting and potentiating, including attention

---

* Since writing this, the authors have learned by personal communication that Drs. Ernest Sachs, Jr. and Donald Wilson have done essentially this procedure on two tic patients at Hanover, New Hampshire. Both patients reportedly had relief of their tic pain.

phenomena and abnormal psychic states such as anxiety and depression. Temporal input factors and central repetitive neuron discharges have yet to be fully integrated into a comprehensive spacial model that is satisfactory to explain all present findings.

In "idiopathic" primary trigeminal neuralgia, the pathological etiological factors increasingly appear to be peripheral in many cases (2, 32); and, these pathologies are probably varied in both cause and location. In those cases presently accepted by all as "symptomatic" trigeminal neuralgia, there does appear still to be a disproportionate percentage involving pathology at the posterior root level as Dandy noted long ago. These peripheral abnormalities secondarily establish in certain individuals with presumed central prerequisites (such as neuron "drop out" with aging, etc.), *probably by deafferentiation,* or at least by alteration of the normal input frequency code, a hyperactive epileptiform central focus, abnormal insofar as is now known only from a physiological, and hence also a chemical, viewpoint. No "short circuit" due to demyelinization between remaining sensory input fibers and either antidromic sensory potentials or hypothetically postulated parasympathetic efferent fibers needs to be implicated. While in some types of chronic pain, therapeutic measures may include stimulation of competing, or inhibiting, central circuits (i.e. stimulation of low threshold large medulated touch "A" fibers), most neurosurgical procedures for the relief of tic pain can be considered as forms of *further quantitatively and spacially significant deafferentiation* of this hypothetical abnormal hyperactive central focus to a critical level below firing threshold. It can also be viewed as an abolition of the remaining perverted sensory input in the crucial area. Medical therapy at present can be considered as basically anticonvulsant.

In conclusion, it is to be hoped that in the future additional pharmaceutical preparations will be found to give "total" control of pain caused by tic douloureux without surgical intervention. However, until such a time arrives it appears that in some cases of true tic douloureux in which the patient does not respond to Dilantin, Tolseram or Tegretol, or proves allergic, the trigeminal compression procedure still offers a relatively safe operative approach without significant postoperative facial anesthesia.

REFERENCES

1. ALLING, C. C.: *Facial Pain*. Philadelphia Lea & F., 1968.
2. BEAVER, D. L.: Electron microscopy of the gasserian ganglion in trigeminal neuralgia *J Neurosurg (Supplement)*, 26:138, 1967.
3. BECKER, D. P.; GLUCK, H.; NULSEN, F. E., and JANE, J. A.: An inquiry into the neurophysiological basis for pain. *J Neurosurg*, 30:1, 1969.

4. BLOOM, S.: Tic douloureux treated with new anticonvulsant. *Arch Neurol (Chicago),* 9:285, 1963.

5. CARREGAL, E. J. A.; AGNEW, W. F.; CRUE, B. L., and TODD, E. M.: Tolseram—Effect on trigeminal antidromic potentials. *Bull Los Angeles Neurol Soc,* 30:216, 1965.

6. CARREGAL, E. J. A.; CRUE, B. L., and TODD, E. M.: Further observation of trigeminal antidromic potentials. Possible physiological function of sensory antidromic potentials. *J Neurosurg,* 20:277, 1963.

7. CASEY, K. L., and MELZAK, R.: Neural mechanisms of pain: A conceptual model. In Way, E. L. (Ed.): *New Concepts in Pain and Its Clinical Management.* Philadelphia, Davis, 1967.

8. CHINITZ, A.; SEELINGER, D. F., and GREENHOUSE, A. H.: Anticonvulsant therapy in trigeminal neuralgia. *Amer J Med Sci,* 252:62, 1966.

9. CRUE, B. L., and CARREGAL, E. J. A.: Neuralgia as central pain. *Excerpta Medica,* 36:E 66, 1961.

10. CRUE, B. L., CARREGAL, E. J. A., and TODD, E. M.: Neuralgia—Discussion of central mechanisms. *Bull Los Angeles Neurol Soc,* 29:107, 1964.

11. CRUE, B. L.; KILHAM, O.; CARREGAL, E. J. A., and TODD, E. M.: Peripheral trigeminal potentials. *Bull Los Angeles Neurol Soc,* 32:17, 1967.

12. CRUE, B. L.; SHELDEN, C. H.; PUDENZ, R. H., and FRESHWATER, D. B.: Observations on the pain and trigger mechanisms in trigeminal neuralgia. *Neurology (Minneap),* 6:196, 1956.

13. CRUE, B. L., and SUTIN, J.: Trigeminal nerve potentials and their relation to tic douloureux, *J Neurosurg,* 16:477, 1959.

14. CRUE, B. L., and TODD, E. M.: Trigeminal neuralgia. *Curr Diag,* 728, 1968.

15. CRUE, B. L., and TODD, E. M.: Vagal neuralgia. In Vinken, P. J., and Bruyn, G. W. (Eds.): *Handbook of Clinical Neurology,* vol. 5. Amsterdam, North Holland Publishing Co., 1968.

16. CRUE, B. L.; TODD, E. M., and CARREGAL, E. J. A.: Posterior approach for percutaneous cervical cordotomy. *Confin Neurol,* 30:41, 1968.

17. CRUE, B. L.; TODD, E. M., and CARREGAL, E. J. A.: Cranial neuralgia—neurophysiological considerations. In Vinken, P. J., and Bruyn, G. W. (Eds): *Handbook of Clinical Neurology,* vol. 5. Amsterdam, North Holland Publishing Co., 1968.

18. CRUE, B. L.; TODD, E. M.; CARREGAL, E. J. A., and KILHAM, O.: Percutaneous trigeminal tractotomy. *Bull Los Angeles Neurol Soc,* 32:87, 1967.

19. CRUE, B. L., TODD, E. M., and DUEMLER, L. P.: Pain as sensory epilepsy. *Bull Los Angeles Neurol Soc,* 32:33, 1967.

20. CRUE, B. L.; TODD, E. M., and LOEW, A. G.: Tolseram—Clinical use in trigeminal neuralgia. *Bull Los Angeles Neurol Soc,* 30:212, 1965.

21. DARIAN-SMITH, I., and YOKOTA, T.: Cortically evoked depolarization of trigeminal cutaneous afferent fibers in the cat. *J Neurophysiol,* 29:170, 1966.

22. ECCLES, J. C.: *The Physiology of Synapsis.* Berlin, Springer, 1964.

23. FRANZ, D. N., and IGGO, A.: Dorsal root potentials and ventral root reflexes evoked by nonmyelinated fibers. *Science,* 162:1140, 1968.

24. FROMM, G. H., and KILLIAN, J. M.: Effect of some anticonvulsant drugs on the spinal trigeminal nucleus. *Neurology (Minneap),* 17:275, 1967.

25. GARDNER, J.: Trigeminal neuralgia. *Clin Neursurg,* 15:1, 1968.

26. GARDNER, W. J., and PINTO, J. P.: The Taarnhoj operation: Relief of trigeminal neuralgia without numbness. *Cleveland Clin Quart,* 20:364, 1953.

27. GRAY, E. G.: A morphological basis for pre-synaptic inhibition? *Nature (London)*, 193:82, 1962.

28. IANNONE, A.; BAKER, A. B., and MORRELL, F.: Dilantin in the treatment of trigeminal neuralgia. *Neurology (Minneap)*, 8:126, 1958.

29. JANNETTA, P. J., and RAND, R. W.: Transtentorial retrogasserian rhizotomy in trigeminal neuralgia by microneurosurgical technique. *Bull Los Angeles Neurol Soc*, 31:93, 1966.

30. KELLY, M.: Is pain due to pressure on nerves? *Neurology (Minneap)*, 6:32, 1956.

31. KERR, F. W. L.: Ultra structure of the spinal tract of the trigeminal nerve and the substantia gelatinosa. *Exp Neurol*, 16:359, 1966.

32. KERR, F. W. L.: Correlated light and electron microscopic observations on the normal trigeminal ganglion and sensory root in man. *J Neurosurg (Supplement)*, 26:132, 1967.

33. KING, B. R.: The medical control of tic douloureux. Preliminary report of the effect of mephenesin on facial pain. *J Neurosurg*, 15:290, 1958.

34. KING, R. B.: The value of mephenesin carbamate in the control of pain in patients with tic douloureux. *J Neurosurg*, 25:153, 1966.

35. KING, R. B.: Evidence for a central etiology of tic douloureux. *J Neurosurg (Supplement)*, 26:175, 1967.

36. KING, R. B., and BARNETT, J. C.: Studies of trigeminal nerve potentials. Overreaction to tactile facial stimulation in acute laboratory preparations. *J Neurosurg*, 14:617, 1957.

37. KING, R. B., and MEAGHER, J. N.: Studies of trigeminal nerve potentials. *J Neurosurg*, 12:393, 1955.

38. KING, R. B.; MEAGHER, J. N., and BARNETT, J. C.: Studies of trigeminal nerve potentials in normal compared to abnormal experimental preparations. *J Neurosurg*, 13:176, 1956.

39. KRUGER, L.: Structural aspects of trigeminal neuralgia: A summary of current findings and concepts. *J Neurosurg (Supplement)*, 26:109, 1967.

40. LIVINGSTON, R. B.: Central control of afferent activity. In Jasper, H. H. *et al.* (Eds.): *Henry Ford Hospital International Symposium. Reticular Formation of the Brain.* Boston, Little, 1958.

41. MAMO, H., and LOGET, P.: Une manifestation neurophysiologique paradoxole, le reflex antidromique sensitivo-sensitif de Toennies. *Rev Franc Biol*, February, 1958.

42. MELZAK, R., and WALL, P. D.: Pain mechanisms: A new theory. *Science*, 150:971, 1965.

43. MELZAK, R., and WALL, P. D.: Gate control theory of pain. In Soulaerac, A.; Cahn, J., and Charpentier, J. (Eds.) *Pain.* New York, Academic, 1968, p. 11.

44. NASHOLD, B. S., and WILSON, W. P.: Central pain observations in man with chronic implanted electrodes in the midbrain tegmentum. *Confin Neurol*, 27:30, 1966.

45. NASHOLD, JR., B. S.; WILSON, W. P., and SLOUGHTER, D. G.: Sensations evoked by stimulation in the midbrain of man. *J Neurosurg*, 30:14, 1969.

46. NASHOLD, JR., B. S.; WILSON, W. P., and SLOUGHTER, D. G.: Stereotaxic midbrain lesions for central dysesthesia and phantom pain. *J Neurosurg*, 30:116, 1969.

47. PENMAN, J.: Trigeminal neuralgia. In Vinken, P. J., and Bruyn, G. W. (Eds.): *Handbook of Clinical Neurology*, vol. 5. Amsterdam, North Holland Publishing Co., 1967.

48. REXED, B.: The cytoarchitectonic organization of the spinal cord in the cat. *J Comp Neurol*, 96:415, 1952.

49. SHEALEY, C. N.; MORTIMER, J. T., and RESWICK, J. B.: Electrical inhibition of pain by stimulation of the dorsal columns. *Anesth Analg (Cleveland)*, 46:489, 1967.

50. SHEALY, C. N.; TASHTY, N.; MORTIMER, J. T., and BECKER, D. P.: Electrical inhibition of pain: Experimental evaluation. *Anesth Analg (Cleveland)*, 46:299, 1967.

51. SHELDEN, C. H.; CRUE, B. L., and COULTER, J. A.: Surgical treatment of trigeminal neuralgia and discussion of compression operation. *Postgrad Med*, 27:595, 1960.

52. SHELDEN, C. H.; PUDENZ, R. H., and DOYLE, J.: Electrical control of facial pain. *Amer J Surg*, 114:209, 1967.

53. SHELDEN, C. H.; PUDENZ, R. H.; FRESHWATER, D. B., and CRUE, B. L.: Compression rather than decompression for trigeminal neuralgia. *J Neurosurg*, 12:123, 1956.

54. SHENDE, M. C., and KING, R. B.: Excitability changes of trigeminal primary afferent preterminals in brain stem nuclear complex of squirrel monkey. *J Neurophysiol*, 30:949, 1967.

55. STERNBACH, R. A.: *Pain—A Psychophysiological Analysis*. New York, Academic, 1968.

56. STEWART, W. A., and KING, R. B.: A new ascending spinal trigeminal neural pathway. *Surg Forum*, 12:386, 1961.

57. STEWART, W. A., and KING, R. B.: Fiber projections from the nucleus candalis of the spinal trigeminal nucleus. *J Comp Neurol*, 121:271, 1963.

58. STEWART, D. H., and KING, R. B.: Effect of conditioning stimuli upon evoked potentials in the trigeminal complex. *J Neurophysiol*, 29:443, 1966.

59. STEWART, W. A.; STOOPS, W. L., and KING, R. B.: Trigeminal dorsal root reflex. *Surg Forum*, 14:405, 1963.

60. STEWART, W. A.; STOOPS, W. L.; PILLARRE, P. R., and KING, R. B.: An electrophysiologic study of ascending pathways from nucleus candalis of the trigeminal nucleus complex. *J Neurosurg*, 19:35, 1964.

61. STOOKEY, B., and RAUSOHOFF, J.: *Trigeminal Neuralgia*. Springfield, Thomas, 1959.

62. SWEET, W. H.: Pain. In Field, J.; Magoun, H. W., and Hall, V. E. (Eds.): *Handbook of Physiology*. Washington, D.C., American Physiol. Soc., 1959.

63. SZENTAGOTHAI, J.: Neuronal and synaptic arrangements in the substantial gelatinosa. *J Comp Neurol*, 122:219, 1964.

64. TAARNHOJ, P.: Decompression of the trigeminal root and the posterior part of the ganglion as treatment in trigeminal neuralgia. *J Neurosurg*, 9:288, 1952.

65. TODD, E. M.; CRUE, B. L., and VERGODAMO, M.: Conservative treatment of postherpetic neuralgia. *Bull Los Anegeles Neurol Soc*, 30:148, 1965.

66. TORVALIS, A.: Sensory, motor and reflex changes in two cases of intractable pain after stereotactic mesencephalic tractotomy. *J Neurol Neurosurg Psychiat*, 22:299, 1959.

67. TURNBULL, I. M.; BLACK, R. G., and SCOTT, J. W.: Reflex efferent impulses in the trigeminal nerve. *J Neurosurg*, 17:746, 1961.

68. WALL, P. D.: Repetitive discharge of neurons. *J Neurophysiol*, 22:305, 1959.

69. WALL, P. D.: Presynaptic control of impulses at the first central synapse in the cutaneous pathway. In Eccles, J. C., and Schade, J. P. (Eds.): *Progress in Brain Research*. Amsterdam, Elsevier, 1964.

70. WALL, P. D., and SWEET, W. H.: Temporary abolition of pain in man. *Science*, 155:108, 1967.

71. WHITE, J. C., SWEET, W. H.: *Pain—Its Mechanisms and Neurosurgical Control*. Springfield, Thomas, 1955.

72. WOLTMAN, H. W.; WILLIAMS, H. L., and LAMBERT, E. H.: An attempt to relieve

hemifacial spasm by neurolysis of the facial nerves. *Proc Mayo Clinic,* 26:236, 1951.

73. WYKE, B.: The neurology of facial pain. *Brit J Hosp Med,* 1:46, 1968.
74. ZIMMERMAN, M.: Dorsal root potentials after C-fiber stimulation. *Science,* 160:896, 1968.

Chapter 8

COMPRESSION OF INTRACRANIAL PORTION OF FACIAL NERVE AND SECTION OF NERVUS INTERMEDIUS FOR HEMIFACIAL SPASM

BENJAMIN L. CRUE, JR., EDWIN M. TODD AND ENRIQUE J. A. CARREGAL

HEMIFACIAL spasm is a rare clinical entity of unknown etiology with no generally accepted treatment. The presently proposed method of surgical treatment of patients with this motor disorder has been presented previously (3, 5). Classical hemifacial spasm is usually unaccompanied by pain and is unrelated to geniculate neuralgia (7, 10). On occasion, it may be associated with true tic pain, the so-called "tic convulsif." The hemifacial spasm, even when painless, often causes considerable psychological suffering to the individual afflicted. Available evidence tends to indicate that there is a nuclear basis for the clonic spasms (1). The relationship between primary trigeminal neuralgia (tic douloureux) and hemifacial spasm has been discussed by Gardner (9). It has been postulated that the underlying mechanism in trigeminal neuralgia involves central epileptiform discharge, i.e., sensory epilepsy of central neuron aggregates (2). An analogous mechanism has been proposed for hemifacial spasm, independent of any possible peripheral etiology, as a form of localized epilepsy limited to the unilateral 7th motor nucleus (4). Accordingly, if partial deafferentation by the compression procedure on the trigeminal posterior root is effective treatment in trigeminal neuralgia, it may be that a compression procedure on the intracranial portion of the 7th cranial nerve might be efficacious in treating patients who have hemifacial spasm, with proper care being taken to avoid damaging the nerves sufficiently to cause a Bell's palsy. Moreover, the 7th nerve being mainly motor, intriguing additional advantages are conceivable from section of the nervus intermedius to reduce afferent inflow into this region and perhaps to modify any trigger mechanism firing the hypothetical epileptiform focus in the region of the 7th nerve nucleus.

Selective and exclusive section of the nervus intermedius (11) would probably not be effective. This is demonstrated by the fact that local anesthetics in the middle ear do not decrease the movement of hemifacial spasm. Alternatively, procedures concerned solely with the 7th motor nerve have not sufficed short of total destruction of the nerve. In these cases resolution of the inevitable Bell's palsy with return of voluntary motor activity has reportedly been associated with reactivation of involuntary hemifacial spasms in many patients. Retrospective analysis of the unfavorable background of each of these procedures done separately led to speculation regarding a combined approach. Section of the nervus intermedius intracranially, with simultaneous gentle compression of the 7th nerve, utilizing a posterior fossa approach to the cerebellar pontine angle was proposed. This was first carried out by the authors in 1961, and in the subsequent eight years the procedure has been performed in a total of five patients with hemifacial spasm.

There was immediate cessation of hemifacial spasm without significant Bell's palsy in all five cases. So far there have been two recurrences. This is an unsatisfactory 40 percent recurrence rate. One woman operated upon in 1962 had two recurrences, necessitating repeat intracranial operations. This culminated in Bragdon's procedure of crushing the 7th nerve, deliberately giving a Bell's palsy. The patient has subsequently been lost to follow-up. She died of acute coronary thrombosis at home two and one-half years after the initial surgery. Another woman had a recurrence, and three years later, in 1965, had an electronic blocking device installed peripherally by Dr. C. H. Shelden. In the three remaining patients there has been no recurrence after follow-up from one to eight years.

The belief that hemifacial spasm may be an epileptic disorder perhaps gains further support from the observation that in four cases over this same period of time (i.e., in about one case out of six where it has been tried), diphenyl hydantoin (Dilantin), gr 1½, q.i.d., has had a significant effect in abolishing or decreasing the involuntary movements of hemifacial spasm. No other medication, including several different anticonvulsants, has been effective. Surgical intervention has remained the procedure of last resort, and only in those patients so severely afflicted that surgery of a major nature seemed justified. Of the five patients operated upon, four were women who had found the cosmetic defect of hemifacial spasm psychologically intolerable. One patient was a man, a research entomologist, who found that the hemifacial spasm interfered with his work, which required use of a microscope.

The most recent craniotomy was performed utilizing the Zeiss binocular operative microscope. In none of the five cases was a significant abnormality found in the cerebellar pontine angle at surgery. Specifically, no unusual loop of the internal auditory artery was found that appeared grossly to be in any way playing an etiological role. This is contrary to the report of others (8). The authors, therefore, can make no comments concerning the occurrence of peripheral versus central pathology to explain the etiology of hemifacial spasm. Yet, it must be recorded that,

analogous to trigeminal neuralgia, it is entirely possible to have a peripheral etiology initiating an abnormal physiological central mechanism, at
least in theory.

The relationship of the trigeminal nerve to hemifacial spasm has been
of interest (9). As reported previously (4), in one case of nonpainful
hemifacial spasm, an intraorbital block in the 2nd trigeminal division decreased, but did not stop, the hemifacial spasm on the afflicted side. In
one case of tic convulsif, i.e. hemifacial spasm associated with true tic pain
on the ipsilateral side, a trigeminal compression procedure performed by
Dr. D. B. Freshwater through the middle fossa alleviated the pain but
failed to stop permanently the motor movements of the hemifacial spasm,
which recurred shortly following surgery.

The operation of posterior fossa craniotomy for exploration of the
cerebellar pontine angle is certainly a major undertaking. Yet with modern anesthesia and surgical techniques, it is not a difficult operation. It
must be mentioned that in one of the five cases mentioned in this report,
postoperative total deafness resulted on the operated side (in this case
due entirely to inadvertent and unintentional trauma to the 8th nerve).
The risk of hearing loss postoperatively has recently been emphasized by
Scoville (14). The nervus intermedius can usually be separated grossly
(12, 13) from between the 7th and 8th cranial nerves, lifted up with a
blunt hook and sectioned. (See Fig. 8-1.) It is extremely difficult, however, to section the nervus intermedius with certainty without doing at
least some exploration around the 7th nerve. Thus, intracranial section
of nervus intermedius in hemifacial spasm without some degree of trauma
(whether considered a compression or decompression) to the facial nerve
has not been reported. Whether section of the nervus intermedius in the
middle ear by an otolaryngologist, raising a flap in the tympanic membrane, would offer any advantages over local injection through the ear
drum or over local cocainization of Meckel's ganglion (6), must also be
considered in the future. At present, the value of the addition of nervus
intermedius section to the procedure of facial compression in the treatment of hemifacial spasm remains entirely hypothetical and unproven.

At this time there can be no definite answer as to whether facial compression, as carried out by the authors, is truly an effective operation.
This must be determined by further study of a larger series of cases.
Also unanswered is the question as to whether this procedure is at least
temporarily effective, even in this small series, because of the mechanism
of compression as hypothesized by the authors, or whether there is subsequent edema and an internal neurolysis, i.e., a decompression and a
breaking up of any possible etiological short circuits, as proposed by

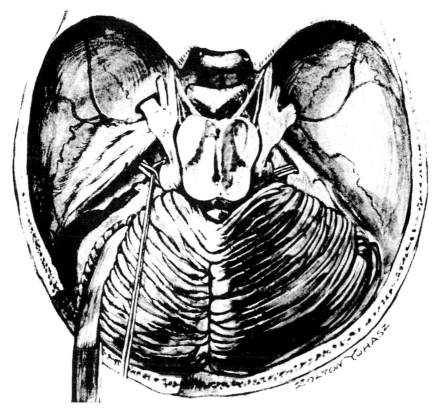

Figure 8-1. Drawing of the intracranial approach to the cerebellar pontine angle, with elevation of nervus intermedius by blunt hook prior to sectioning and prior to gentle compression of the intracranial portion of the facial nerve (from movie—see (3)).

Gardner (9). It does appear that in those few cases of severe hemifacial spasm in which the patient is unable to tolerate the condition and in which major operative intervention seems indicated, then perhaps section of the nervus intermedius and gentle compression of the intracranial portion of the 7th nerve is superior to the crushing of the 7th nerve with the disfiguring and often poorly tolerated Bell's palsy as inevitable sequelae. Thus, the compression procedure for the 7th cranial nerve certainly deserves further investigation and clinical trial, although the recurrence rate may prove unacceptable in the long run.

REFERENCES

1. CAWTHORN, T.: Clonic facial spasm. *Arch Otolaryng*, 81:504, 1965.
2. CRUE, B. L.; SHELDEN, C. H.; PUDENZ, R. H., and FRESHWATER, D. B.: Observations on the pain and trigger mechanism in trigeminal neuralgia. *Neurology (Minneap)*, 6:196, 1956.

 3. CRUE, B. L.; CARREGAL, E. J. A.; SHELDEN, C. H.; PUDENZ, R. H., and TODD, E. M.:
    Intracranial compression of the facial nerve for treatment of facial hemispasm
    (Movie). Presented at the 14th Annual Conference of the Southern California
    Neurological Society, Pebble Beach, California, 1962.
 4. CRUE, B. L.; CARREGAL, E. J. A., and TODD, E. M.: Neuralgia—Consideration of
    central mechanisms. *Bull Los Angeles Neurol Soc*, 29:128, 1964.
 5. CRUE, B. L.; TODD, E. M., and CARREGAL, E. J. A.: Compression of intracranial por-
    tion of facial nerve and section of nervus intermedius for hemifacial spasm. *Bull
    Los Angeles Neurol Soc*, 33:70, 1968.
 6. DYSART, B. R.: Modern view of neuralgia referable to Meckel's ganglion. *Arch
    Otolaryng*, 40:29, 1944.
 7. FURLOW, L. T.: Tic douloureux of the nervus intermedius. *JAMA*, 119:255, 1942.
 8. GARDNER, W. J., and SAVA, G. A.: Hemifacial spasm—A reversible pathophysiological
    state. *J Neurosurg*, 19:240, 1962.
 9. GARDNER, W. J.: Concerning the mechanism of trigeminal neuralgia and hemifacial
    spasm. *J Neurosurg*, 19:947, 1962.
10. HUNT, J. R.: Geniculate neuralgia. *Arch Neurol Psychiat*, 37:253, 1937.
11. PUDENZ, R. H.; SHELDEN, C. H., and KINGMAN, A. F.: Section of the nervus inter-
    medius. Presented to the Southern California Neurosurgical Society, Pebble Beach,
    Calif., 1952.
12. RHOTAN, A. L., JR.; SHIGEAHI, K., and HOLLENSHEAD, W. H.: Nervus intermedius.
    J Neurosurg, 29:609, 1968.
13. SACHS, E., JR.: The role of the nervus intermedius in facial neuralgia. *J Neurosurg*,
    28:54, 1968.
14. SCOVILLE, W. B.: Hearing loss following exploration of cerebello-pontine angle in
    treatment of hemifacial spasm. *J Neurosurg* (in press).

Chapter 9

PERCUTANEOUS RADIOFREQUENCY STEREOTAXIC TRIGEMINAL TRACTOTOMY

Benjamin L. Crue, Jr., Edwin M. Todd and Enrique J. A. Carregal

A TECHNIQUE for percutaneous trigeminal tractotomy was described by the authors in 1967 (2). A total of six patients have undergone this operation, utilizing this stereotaxic radiofrequency technique (12). Four of the patients were treated for neoplastic disease and two for primary trigeminal neuralgia. There were four satisfactory results, one fair result and one failure.

The basic operation of trigeminal tractotomy was introduced by Sjoqvist in 1937 (9). Some surgeons, such as Raney *et al.* (6), have further modified this open operation. Most surgeons, however, consider the posterior fossa craniotomy necessary for the approach to be too major an undertaking, especially when compared with the subtemporal extradural operation for tic douloureux. Tractotomy in the brain stem has done much to provide information about the intriguing anatomy and neurophysiology of this area. Recently, Kunc has reported selective tractotomy for essential glossopharyngeal neuralgia (4). That the upper cervical area could be attacked percutaneously has been well documented by Mullan *et al.* (5) and Rosomoff *et al.* (7, 8).

As stereotaxic equipment improved over earlier, simpler models (11), it appeared that a stereotaxic approach to the lower brain stem might be feasible even in man. The trigeminal region in the lower medulla was approached posteriorly in the cat in the laboratory, and excellent localization could be obtained by monitoring the evoked responses to infraorbital nerve stimulation (Fig. 9-1). In the human being, initial attempts to approach the descending trigeminal nucleus and tract stereotaxically through an electrode inserted in a manner similar to a cisternal needle puncture were carried out in the morgue. It proved possible to introduce an electrode angled slightly upward above the arch of C1 and below the posterior rim of the foramen magnum, slightly lateral to the midline, so as to enter the area of the trigeminal tract and nucleus. The target area is illustrated in Figure 9-2. In the cadaver, the needle puncture always appeared to be slightly caudad to the obex; and, so far, both in the morgue and in the six human patients, the posterior-inferior cerebellar artery has not been encountered. Cross sections of several medullae at this

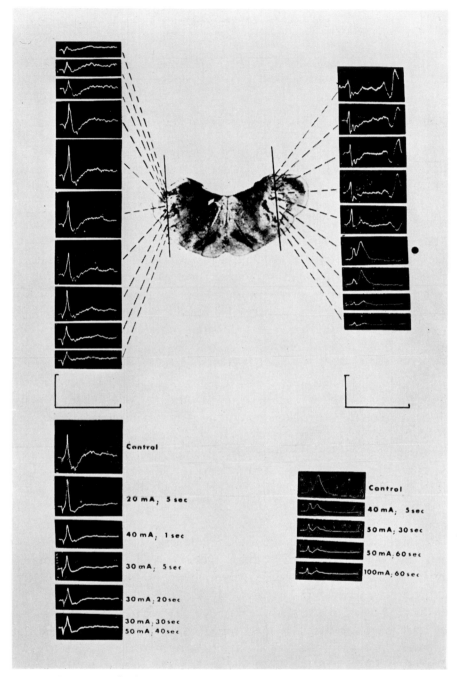

Figure 9-1. A cat anesthetized with sodium pentobarbital, i.p., 30 mg/kg, was placed in the Wells animal stereotaxic instrument. A steel needle electrode (gauge 22) was inserted gradually through a small parietal bony defect aiming at the descending trigeminal complex. The records as illustrated were taken at successive depths following

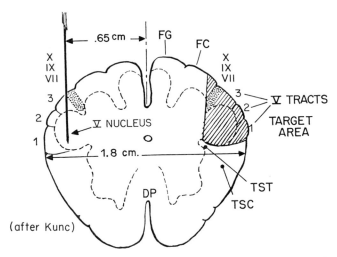

Figure 9-2. Diagrammatic cross section of brain stem at target level (after Kunc, [4]).

level give a rather uniform width of approximately 18 mm. An arbitrary point of 6.5 mm from the midline was selected for initial trial. The estimation of midline was based on the assumption that the midline of the lower medulla and upper cervical cord, with the head and neck in neutral position, should overlay the midline of the odontoid process seen in the posterior-anterior roentgenograph. It is still unproven whether this is a uniformly valid assumption and measurement. It was believed that the radiofrequency (1, 10) lesion should be made approximately 4 mm down

←----

percutaneous stimulation of the ipsilateral infraorbital nerve. As the electrode was being lowered, the size of the evoked response increased until it reached a maximum; thereafter, the response decreased. The electrode was elevated back to the point of maximal response, and at this point a lesion was made by passing a high frequency current between the recording electrode and an indifferent electrode in the ipsilateral temporal muscle. Also illustrated is a transverse section of the brain stem of the cat showing the size and location of the lesions produced. At either side of the section is a series of recordings displaying the response evoked by stimulation of the ipsilateral infraorbital nerve before making the radiofrequency lesion. On the left side, the recordings consist primarily of an early afferent spike, indicating that the electrode is primarily recording from the descending trigeminal tract. On the right side, the recordings consist of a smaller early afferent spike, followed by a transynaptic later response, indicating that the electrode is more medial in the trigeminal nucleus. At the bottom are two series of recordings taken from the point of maximal response, before and after successive lesions, as indicated. Calibration lines represent 10 msec (horizontal) and 1 mV (vertical on the left) and 0.5 mV (vertical on the right). The dot on the right indicates a gain reduction by a factor of 5, i.e., vertical line represents 5 mV, as the needle was lowered initially (2).

from the dorsal surface of the cord (just lateral and caudad to the obex). This has proven to be the most difficult measurement to make. Initial attempts to outline the dorsal surface of the cord, using Pantopaque, have met with failure. So far, in all cases, it has been possible to feel the electrode when it comes in contact with the dorsal surface. Recently, we have utilized impedance monitoring to establish penetration of nervous tissue. Also yet to be tried is the suggestion of Dr. R. Smith, who has advocated injection of tantalum filings to outline by x-ray the anatomy in this area (personal communication).

It was believed that initial clinical attempts should be limited to patients with far-advanced proven malignancy and uncontrolled pain because of the possible hazards of this procedure. However, after the first two patients with neoplasms the authors have treated two patients with primary trigeminal neuralgia (tic douloureux) who were very poor risks for open surgery.

CASE REPORTS

Case 1 (D. S.)

A female, age 56 yrs., had uncontrolled pain in the left periorbital region from carcinoma of the ethmoid sinus. On August 4, 1966, under local anesthesia, the patient was placed prone in the Todd-Wells stereotaxic headpiece and percutaneous trigeminal tractotomy was carried out (2) (Fig. 9-3). X-ray localization was good in the lateral position, but the dorsum of the cord was not outlined by x-ray (Fig. 9-4). The procedure was without incident, and the patient demonstrated postoperatively no untoward reactions. The area of hypalgesia to pinprick is shown in Figure 9-5. This suggests that the lesion was either too ventral or too caudad to have obtained good sensory loss in the third division, but in this particular case with periorbital pain the result was excellent. The patient was relieved subjectively of her pain postoperatively and had a subsequent uneventful demise from her primary disease.

Case 2 (A. B.)

A female 70 yrs., had a sphenoid ridge meningioma for which one of us, in 1959, had done a craniotomy with a Naffziger and Kronelein orbital decompression, followed by a large tantalum cranioplasty. The patient had done well until recent years when she developed increasingly severe periorbital pain not controlled by antidepressants (Elavil) or oral narcotics (Percodan). On May 22, 1967, a similar percutaneous trigeminal tractotomy was carried out. This gave only a relative partial hypalgesia to pinprick over the entire ipsilateral occiput and all three divisions of the trigeminal. However, the pain was, and has remained to the present date,

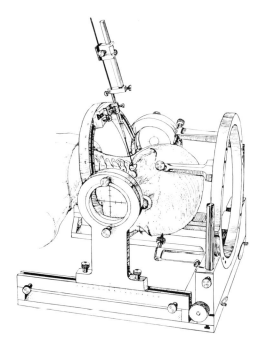

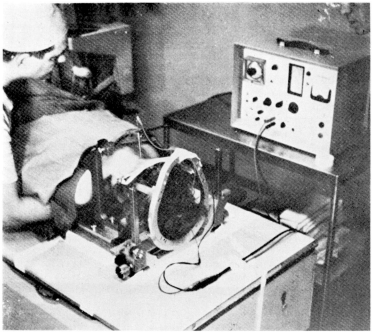

Figure 9-3. *Top:* Drawing of patient's position in Todd-Wells stereotaxic frame for posterior percutaneous trigeminal tractotomy. *Bottom:* Actual patient (prone) with needle in place and electrode in region of left trigeminal tract.

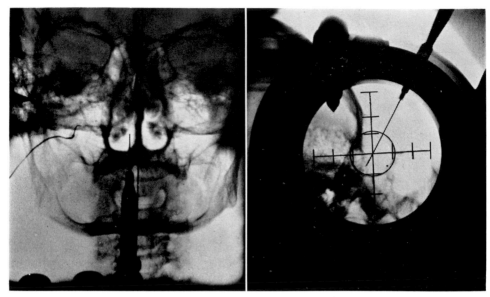

Figure 9-4. X-ray of needle in place (left) lateral view (Polaroid), (right) AP view (Polaroid).

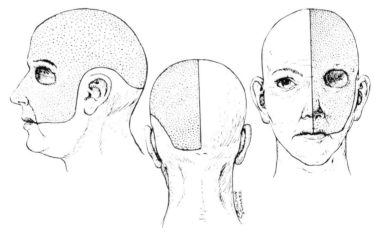

Figure 9-5. Area of postoperative left trigeminal and occipital hypalgesia to pinprick test.

completely relieved. Of interest is the fact that the periorbital edema and conjunctival injection (which almost certainly were due to irritation from the patient's rubbing the area of discomfort) also subsided promptly following the tractotomy and have not recurred. After 2 years there is no significant dysesthesia, although there can be demonstrated some contralateral mild hypalgesia in the trunk and extremities.

Case 3 (S. R.)

A female, 89 yrs., had suffered for a number of years from true tic douloureux of the second division. The patient had proven allergic to Dilantin and had not been relieved by either Tolseram or Tegretol. The patient was in a state of chronic congestive heart failure and had diabetes. In spite of the fact that she did not have a malignancy, she was considered at her age to be in such poor physical condition that open craniotomy was not indicated. On July 11, 1967, she underwent an identical trigeminal tractotomy when infraorbital alcohol injection was not sufficient to stop her pain. Following this procedure the patient also had only a relative hypalgesia to pinprick in all three divisions of the trigeminal and had continued complaints of headache. Nevertheless, her true tic pain disappeared and has not recurred since the tractotomy. Figure 9-6 illustrates how the patient was positioned on the operating table in the surgical suite at the Community Hospital of San Gabriel, where the first five trigeminal tractotomies were carried out. The simul-

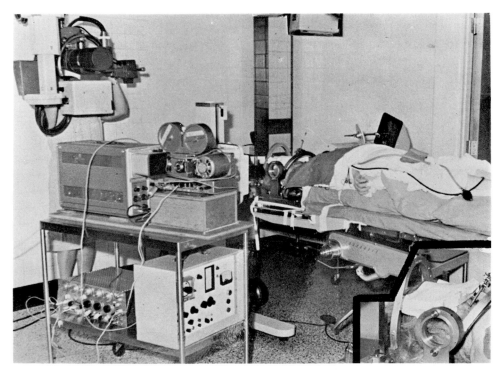

Figure 9-6. Photograph of patient in prone position for posterior approach for percutaneous stereotaxic radiofrequency trigeminal tractotomy in operating room at Community Hospital of San Gabriel. This case is an eighty-nine-year-old woman with second division tic douloureux. (For close-up, see insert lower right.)

taneous biplane x-ray unit was replaced by the small swinging C-arm x-ray unit with an image intensifier which gives an excellent view and allows the surgeons to follow the approach from the lateral aspect. Consequently, only the original PA odontoid alignment necessitates permanent films, and these can be Polaroid films to minimize time.

Case 4 (V. M.)

A male, 51 yrs., was seen because of carcinoma of the base of the tongue. The patient had been treated by surgical intervention and heavy x-irradiation, but was now preterminal because of his inability to eat due to severe unilateral pain in the face and temporomandibular region. A percutaneous trigeminal tractotomy was carried out on December 20, 1968. Postoperatively, the patient had hypalgesia in the first and third division of the ipsilateral trigeminal, with relative sparing of the second division. He had much denser sensory loss over the occipital region. However, the patient was pleased, as the subjective pain was markedly decreased. Over the ensuing months the patient's pain has, unfortunately, again increased in intensity. The patient has had a number of serious hemorrhages in the tumor area and is psychologically depressed and unable or unwilling to come to the office. This must be classified only as a fair result at best.

Case 5 (L. B.)

A female, 86 yrs., had trigeminal neuralgia. The tic complaint was almost incidental, as the patient was in the hospital originally for a large retroperitoneal lymphoma that was biopsied. She was treated by chemotherapy and x-irradiation. Postoperatively, the patient did well except for the continued tic douloureux. The patient did not respond to Tegretol or Tolseram and also appeared allergic to Dilantin. Alcohol blocks were done of both the second and third division, with good areas of analgesia, but there was no relief from the severe true tic pain. It was believed justified to attempt percutaneous tractotomy instead of craniotomy on this patient in view of her age and known intra-abdominal malignancy. Consequently, on December 20, 1968, percutaneous trigeminal tractotomy was attempted. Unfortunately, this patient had cervical osteoarthritis with considerable lordosis of the cervical spine, and it required the needle in an upright position similar to the cordotomy approach (3) to get the electrode between the arch of C1 and the base of the skull. The electrode did hit the bone and was deflected, so that on the first attempt the electrode went lateral to the brain stem and nervous system tissue was not encountered. The electrode and needle were removed and a second approach was made more medially. This appeared to be too far medial, and the small radiofrequency lesions that were placed gave no relief of pain or hypalgesia in the face or occiput. Consequently, the needle was again

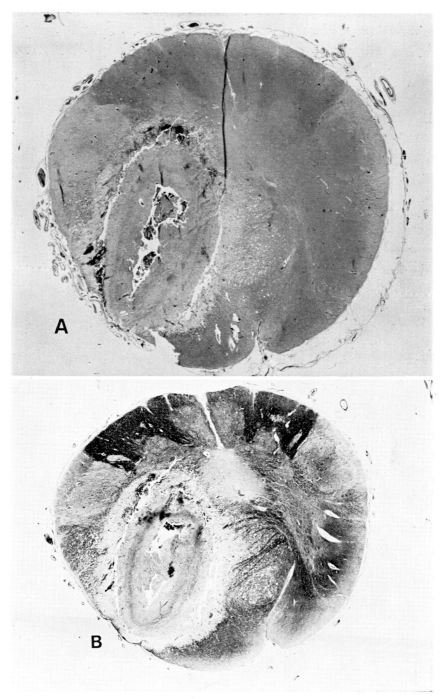

Figure 9-7. Cross section of brain stem patient #6 showing site of maximum stereotaxic radiofrequency lesion, 8 mm caudal to obex. (A) Hematoxylin-eosin stain. (B) Luxol stain for myelin and neurones.

removed. By this time the spinal fluid appeared grossly bloody. The percutaneous trigeminal tractotomy attempt was discontinued. Gratifyingly, and surprisingly, the patient postoperatively had no untoward symptoms other than a mildly stiff neck and some occipital headache. Three days later the patient underwent, in the sitting position, the standard subtemporal craniotomy and had a total posterior root section with relief from her intractable tic pain. This case has to be considered a total failure as far as the percutaneous trigeminal tractotomy is concerned.

Case 6 (L. C.)

A female, 71 yrs., had undergone multiple previous surgical procedures for cylindromatous carcinoma of the soft palate. Finally, the floor of the right middle fossa was eroded and the presence of tumor was determined by brain scan. This appeared to invade the right temporal lobe area. Right facial pain was severe, and after several months was no longer controlled by Triavil and Percodan. The patient developed right total ophthalmoplegia and lost the vision in her right eye. On May 7, 1969, at the City of Hope, a right percutaneous trigeminal tractotomy was performed under very heavy sedation in this preterminal patient. Two lesions were made using 100 miliamps for 30 seconds at depths of 3 and 5 mm as determined by impedance monitoring. A good area of postoperative anesthesia was obtained in the right side of the face and entire head area. No motor weakness or other complication was noted. There was a mild ipsilateral hemihypalgesia. The patient went slowly downhill and expired ten days later. See Figure 9-7. The lesion appears too large, too medial and too deep.

DISCUSSION

While patients with trigeminal neuralgia (tic douloureux) are now responding in a large majority of cases to drug therapy, and while trigeminal subtotal rhizotomy, or root compression, seems effective in managing most of the remaining cases, there are still those patients with pain in the region of the head and neck who require surgical intervention of a more radical nature. In the four patients with invasive neoplasm presented in this paper, it is believed that prior to percutaneous trigeminal tractotomy they might well have had to undergo posterior fossa craniotomy, in spite of their precarious condition. It would appear that there is still a place in the neurosurgeon's armamentarium for either trigeminal tractotomy or total section of the trigeminal root plus nervus intermedius, 9th, and upper portion of the 10th cranial nerve. It is believed justifiable to run some risk in perfecting a safe percutaneous stereotaxic procedure if it obviates the need for such major surgery. However, the authors wish to state unequivocally that, in their opinion, percutaneous trigeminal tractotomy is still in an experimental stage and much further experience is necessary before it can be considered to be acceptably safe or that uniformly satisfactory clinical results may be obtained by means of this technique.

A secondary benefit expected from percutaneous stereotaxic trigeminal tractotomy was the opportunity to obtain neurophysiological recordings from the human brain stem prior to making the radiofrequency lesions. This has been attempted in all six cases, and some records have been obtained. Their quality compares very poorly to tracings from the laboratory animal, and no useful purpose would be served by using any of these records for illustration. So far, the use of evoked potentials in the human trigeminal nerve like those used in the cat has not even proven satisfactory in facilitating localization of the electrode prior to making the lesions. It is hoped that in the near future by using long but smaller concentric bipolar electrodes and a computer averaging technique that recordings can be improved.

It was expected that there might be more spontaneous repetitive activity in the central trigeminal system or more prolonged activity after potentials following evoking stimuli in the tic patients than in cancer patients. This has not been substantiated and the hypothesis is as yet unverified.

REFERENCES

1. BRODKEY, J. S.; MIYAZAKI, Y.; ERVIN, F. R., and MARK, V. H.: Reversible heat lesions with radiofrequency current. *J Neurosurg,* 21:49, 1964.
2. CRUE, B. L.; TODD, E. M.; CARREGAL, E. J. A., and KILHAM, O.: Percutaneous trigeminal tractotomy—Case report utilizing stereotactic radiofrequency lesions. *Bull Los Aangeles Neurol Soc,* 32:86, 1967.
3. CRUE, B. L.; TODD, E. M., and CARREGAL, E. J. A.: Posterior approach for high cervical percutaneous radiofrequency cordotomy. *Confin Neurol,* 30:41, 1968.
4. KUNC, Z.: Treatment of essential neuralgia of the IXth nerve by selective tractotomy. *J Neurosurg,* 23:494, 1965.
5. MULLAN, S.; HARPER, P. V.; HEKMATPANAH, J.; TORRES, H., and DOBBIN, G.: Percutaneous interruption of spinal pain-tracts by means of a strontium 90 needle. *J Neurosurg,* 20:931, 1963.
6. RANEY, R.; RANEY, A. A., and HUNTER, C. R.: Treatment of major trigeminal neuralgia through section of the trigeminal tract in the medulla. *Amer J Surg,* 80:11, 1950.
7. ROSOMOFF, H. L.; CARROLL, F.; BROWN, J., and SHEPTAK, P.: Percutaneous radiofrequency cervical cordotomy: Technique. *J Neurosurg,* 23:639, 1965.
8. ROSOMOFF, H. L.; SHEPTAK, P., and CARROL, F.: Modern pain relief: Percutaneous chordotomy. *JAMA,* 196:482, 1966.
9. SJOQUIST, O.: Studies on pain conduction in the trigeminal nerve. *Acta Psychiat Scand,* Supplementum 17, 1938.

10. SWEET, W. H.; MARK, V. H., and HAMLIN, H.: Radiofrequency lesions in the central nervous system of man and cat. *J Neurosurg,* 17:213, 1960.
11. TODD, E. M.; SHELDEN, C. H.; PUDENZ, R. H., and CRUE, B. L.: Surgical management of dyskinesia. *Amer J Surg* 102:263, 1961.
12. TODD, E. M.; CRUE, B. L., and CARREGAL, E. J. A.: Posterior percutaneous tractotomy and cordotomy. *Confin Neurol* (in press).

Chapter 10

STEREOTAXIC SURGERY FOR RELIEF OF PAIN AND SUFFERING

Edwin M. Todd, Benjamin L. Crue, Jr., William H. Wright
and David B. Maline

A BROADENING spectrum of stereotaxic activity relating to the alleviation of pain and suffering is perhaps less a measure of the value or versatility of these procedures than a reflection of the infinite complexities of the problems. Pain continues to defy attempts to define it precisely, but certain clinical syndromes are recognizable, at least to the extent that remedial attention may be directed to specific central nervous system centers or pathways that we have learned to associate with them. Empirical success with stereotaxic measures that alter or obliterate these centers merely emphasizes the paradox of success in areas of meager mechanistic understanding. It is a curious but cogent reality that, indeed, pain relief is accomplished regularly by means of destructive lesions of the brain on rather flimsy conceptual bases. Pertinent to this discussion is the fact that any predetermined point in the head or neck can now be approached with pinpoint accuracy by stereotaxic methods. Moreover, refinement of technique and sophistication of instrumentation over the past two decades have made possible minimal interference with structural relationships along routes of access as specific targets are destroyed with predictable diameters in discretely circumscribed lesions.

The challenge of unsolved neurophysiological aspects of pain unites the stereotaxic surgeon with the basic research scientist in a dynamic process of relating accumulated data from these operations to known or supposed structural and functional involvement. Revelations from carefully conducted studies are seldom unequivocal, sometimes frankly confusing, often contrary to existing opinion, but always of some statistical value in fitting together the innumerable pieces in the enormous puzzle that is pain. That inadvertency—plausible serendipity—played a major role in helping us to find many of the pieces where stereotaxic surgery has been involved does not detract from the overall contribution, and exciting new challenges are inherent in our awareness that the pieces from this great puzzle remain strewn about in a state of disarray, with many key pieces still missing.

There are three distinct anatomical areas that rather naturally sep-

81

arate stereotaxic surgery into spheres of interest, any one of which may
be singularly exclusive for some surgeons, but in which all may dabble
to variable degree with, perhaps, one chief concern. This division is illustrated best in terms of the operative procedures that are employed in
the given areas; namely, encephalotomy, hypophysectomy and chordotomy (with some overlap of interest in the posterior fossa).

Encephalotomy

Human stereotaxic surgery was introduced by Spiegel and Wycis in
1947 (59). Appropriate to the theme of this symposium, their first case
was a woman with severe facial pain unrelieved by conventional surgical
methods. Enduring benefits were obtained by the application of a guided
probe to deep central structures where planned lesions interrupted pain
pathways in the midbrain and dorsomedial nucleus of the thalamus

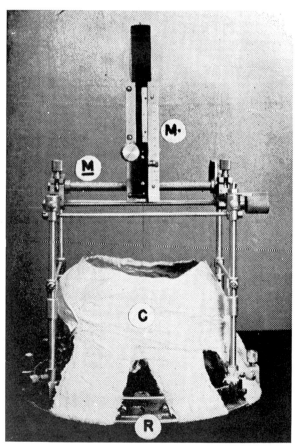

Figure 10-1. Stereoencephalotome: Apparatus used by Spiegel and Wycis for the first
stereotaxic operation on the human brain (59).

(Fig. 10-1) (58). This work stands as a monumental landmark in surgical neurology. Within a remarkably short period, a new subspecies type of neurosurgeon appeared—one who concentrated his interest in and the greater part of his energies on, stereotaxy. Centers rapidly emerged in widespread areas of the world, and the literary outpourings, almost immediately voluminous, became a colossal clutter, still confused but clearing somewhat because of recent organizational efforts. It remains for posterity to sort out the mess of this literary log jam and properly reward original investigation, but it is probably true that circumstances surrounding the blind rush of progress have made it possible for discoveries to occur simultaneously in widely separated centers. For example, confusion continues to exist regarding the first stereotaxic procedure involving the globus pallidus to treat disorders of motion. Introduction of the procedure has been attributed variously to Wycis and Spiegel (69), Narabayashi (49), Riechert (54), Guiot (26), Talairach (62), or Cooper (14). Efforts to assign a singular credit would have to divorce the act from the idea, and the roots of the latter will always be vague.

Controversy erupting in the early 1950's from differences of opinion regarding selection of patients, target sites and modes of lesion-making merely generated more heated discussion to fan the flames of interest and warm the minds of investigators in the remotest corners of the world. Much of the criticism derived from a splintering into factions with opposing viewpoints, the one dedicated to more scientific reliance on neurophysiological data, and the other motivated by grosser clinical empiricism. The dichotomy was, in truth, artificial, because both groups embraced the same basic principles and disagreed only on how much neurophysiological monitoring was *experimental* and how much *practical* for surgical application. The arguments served to emphasize existing shortcomings and stimulated renewed investigative energy (40). By the later 1950's, several significant series had accumulated to clearly establish the impressive advantages in treating patients with disorders of motion and various refractory pain problems (4, 11, 15, 19-21, 25, 34, 39, 40-42, 70). Attempts to alter spasticity and akinesia deficits remain singularly unsuccessful. The outlook for treating patients with epilepsy and severe emotional derangement is bright, but the present is clouded by somewhat capricious preliminary results (7, 22, 30, 47, 63). There is daily reassurance that the ingenuity of the pioneer years is being recapitulated in multiple enterprising centers about the world as a rich variety of new disease entities are critically reappraised in the light of stereotaxic advances (24, 35, 48, 51). Cerebral aneurysm, a most treacherous adversary, has been daringly thrombosed by means of electrical induction (46) and by magnetically controlled metal filings (3). This incorrigible lesion remains the exclusive domain of the superbly qualified. Less spectacular but patently more consequential are some of the developments in basic neuro-physiological orientation.

The fortuitous advent of human stereotaxic surgery in the post World War II era of explosive technological advancement which has provided a rich source of ready scientific knowhow for the emerging specialty is re-flected in the rapid development of sophisticated probing devices and electronic monitoring equipment (5, 45, 60). Microelectrodes gently in-sinuated among delicate central structures for recording, stimulation and potential evocation and tracing have opened new vistas of central nervous system function while supplying pertinent information for immediate practical application to clinical problems (12, 33, 50, 71). Observable ef-fects of stimulation studies have localized elusive target areas in poorly understood structural complexes (2, 9, 27, 28, 37, 67). Impedence changes evidenced by differing cellular densities and fiber tracts encountered by advancing probes offer additional data concerning localization (36). Least understood at this time, but perhaps of greatest potential value, are cur-rent investigations concerned with the recording of spontaneous electrical activity of cells and cell clusters and tracing of potentials along routes of dispersion through the brain (17, 18). The mapping process suffers from want of interpretation at this rudimentary stage, but the enormous por-tent of this infant science in matters of pain, disorder of motion, epilepsy and mental derangement excites the imagination.

Personal experiences with palidotomy and thalmotomy in treating pa-tients with disorders of motion and pain, dating back to 1955, allow a certain latitude for wondrous appraisal of the passing parade (66). It is interesting to recall isolated glories from the crudest methods of chemical destruction, and harpooning techniques which were surprisingly accurate with practice but often nonreproducible (10). One is naturally inclined to forget some of the depressing complications of these early adventures (61). A more penetrating analysis underlines the vast improvement in accuracy and the reduced hazards. Contrasts are all the more striking when projected against the pioneer background.

Today, most medical schools about the world have a subdepartment of stereotaxic surgery, and in this country most neurosurgeons in or out of medical school participate in stereotaxy in some way. There is no uni-versally accepted instrumentation, as many of the more active operators feel a need for highly personalized equipment (6, 44). All modern instru-ments owe a debt of inspiration to the original Horsley-Clarke apparatus (Fig. 10-2) used in animal experimentation during the early years of this century (32). This is true of the Todd-Wells unit used at City of

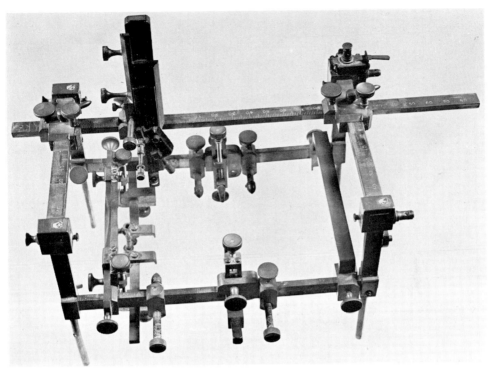

Figure 10-2. Horsley-Clarke Instrument. This is a photograph of the second unit in existence. It was used by Ernest Sachs, Sr., M.D. in Sir Victor Horsley's laboratory in London in 1906 and 1907. Sachs used this instrument when he determined that the thalamus was the central sensory coordinating mechanism rather than a purely optic center as believed previously (56). It was later employed for research activities at Washington University in St. Louis (57) where Sachs held the first professorship and chair in neurological surgery in the world. In a moving ceremony at Yale Medical School in 1956, Sachs donated the instrument to Dr. Horace W. Magoun for permanent investiture at UCLA Medical Center.

Hope Medical Center, and its designers acknowledge variable amounts of petty larceny from all instruments that have preceded it, including those of Talairach (62), Spiegel et al (59), Cooper (16), Rand (53), Guiot (26), Leksell (38), Riechert and Mundinger (55), Bertrand and Martinez (8) and undoubtedly many others.

Suitably ideal to our own special circumstances, a technique has evolved that neatly adapts to a variety of problems, unrelated and anatomically separated, but having a common basis in terms of relieving human suffering. The essence of this particular system of stereotaxic surgery is versatility, in that it allows a range of modifications that encompasses all known stereotaxic routes of access to the head and neck (64). In effect, this simplifies multiple procedural disciplines by minimizing confusion of

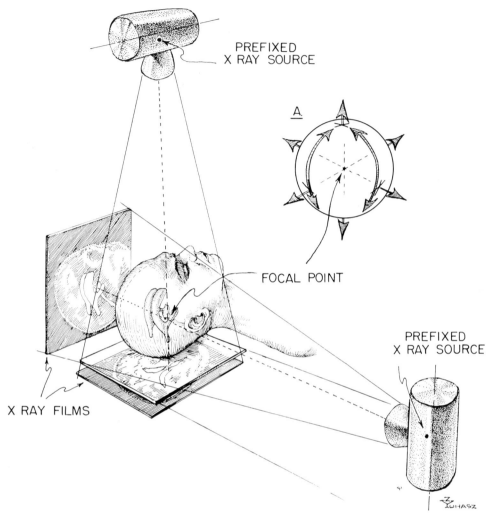

PREFIXED
X RAY SOURCE

A.

FOCAL POINT

PREFIXED
X RAY SOURCE

X RAY FILMS

Figure 10-3. Diagrammatic representation of head positioned for surgery in stereotaxic unit. Inset (A) indicates multidirectional capacity of instrument for moving predetermined target within head to superimpose on preset x-ray convergent point.

participating x-ray and operating room personnel. More important, it expedites operative execution and reduces the chance of mishap or error to a lower denominator. The instrument employed is designed to meet a rigorous requirement for a means of delivering electrodes and other probing devices with microscopic accuracy to any target in the human head or neck. The focal point in this instrument is fixed for the entire system, oriented with the point of convergence of x-ray emissions from permanently stationed x-ray tubes, the lateral ten feet and the AP or PA tube eight feet from the focal point (Fig. 10-3). This relationship is a constant

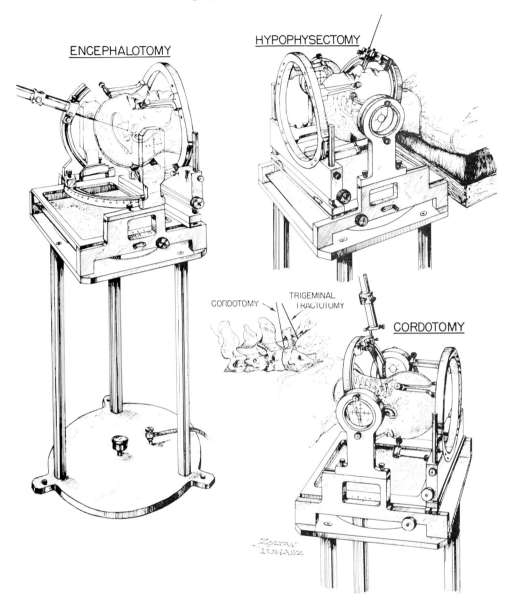

ENCEPHALOTOMY

HYPOPHYSECTOMY

CORDOTOMY ⟍   TRIGEMINAL TRACTOTOMY

CORDOTOMY

Figure 10-4. Composite illustration of stereotaxic procedures described in text. Enlarged detail of upper cervical spine (inset) depicts distinctive sites and angles of entry for posterior percutaneous cordotomy and trigeminal tractotomy.

that permits meaningful analysis of comparative statistics from patient to patient because the focal point, in turn, is always in a fixed position relative to x-ray film. Accordingly, image distortion is always the same and easily correctable to infinity reading on a standard scale for each projection (65). The versatility feature of the instrument is inherent in the fixed focal point, common to both x-rays and instrument, on which the anatomical target can be superimposed with the head or neck in any position for optimal access of probing instrument. The operator is thus enabled to select a route to the anatomical target through structures least likely to be adversely effected by transgressing instrumentation. A preference for radiofrequency methods of producing ultimate lesions emphasizes only one facet of the original intent to provide standardized guides to accommodate all available means of lesion production. In practice, a horizontal quadrant is employed for targets in the neck and posterior fossa and for transnasal hypophysectomy. The vertical quadrant is generally used for supratentorial and upper brain stem objectives. A broader expanse of x-ray picture and more lateral excursion of the vertical fixture make this quadrant more suitable for dealing with certain aspects of epilepsy and emotional problems involving the temporal lobes and paracallosal regions (Fig. 10-4). We have experimented with a portable setup of fixed tubes incorporated into the stereotaxic guide complex, utilizing smaller standard tubes (31) as well as Field Emissions tubes (43), and find the arrangement satisfactory, with little inconvenience other than the matter of properly translating increased image distortion into infinity measurements. Such a setup is endorsed where the tubes used will give adequate definition, provided tube distance is not too confined. Excellent contrast elicited from our distant stationary tube arrangement has discouraged a more vigorous exploration of this alternative, but where facilities are less spacious it is a worthwhile consideration. Our existing stereotaxic method is based upon an eminently flexible system, suitable to all recognized stereotaxic applications at this time. The basic unit is soundly conceived and sufficiently adaptable to serve adequately for any conceivable breakthroughs within the foreseeable future. The mad rush that has characterized the short history of human stereotaxy may be expected to ease somewhat. Horizons are vast but somewhat blurred by the relatively primitive state of knowledge of neurophysiologic mechanisms. Technological advances in instrumentation will continue as needs become evident, and it is entirely justifiable to presume that all existing equipment will be replaced in due time.

Hypophysectomy

Stereotaxic hypophysectomy circumvents the formidable operative obstacles of open cranial surgery by a simple direct transnasal-transsphenoidal route. We have not explored the feasibility of alternative stereotaxic pathways to the sella (23). Our experience has been confined to two thermodestructive methods, i.e., cryogenics and radiofrequency.

Recent cases have been managed exclusively by radiofrequency as a consequence of our conviction that this technique is effective, less time-consuming and inordinately less expensive in terms of generator and probe costs. In all other respects, evaluation of relative merits and disadvantages of radiofrequency and cryogens indicates that they give reasonably comparable results. Our series, in numbers, however, is heavily weighted in favor of radiofrequency. All operations are done under general anesthesia. The relative ease of pre- and postoperative care has extended the criteria of selection to include severely debilitated patients with far-advanced hormone-influenced malignancy, diabetic retinopathy and acromegaly (1, 13, 52, 72). Details of management have been discussed in Chapter 2.

Cordotomy

Percutaneous cordotomy, utilizing principles of stereotaxis to guide lesion-making probes to high cervical targets is a more recent inclusion in the profile of stereotaxic procedures. Yet, in terms of frequency, it is probably the most widely accepted and possibly the most commonly performed stereotaxic procedure at this time in this country. The instant popularity of this technique is attributable to the fact that it represents a vastly simplified means of accomplishing a pain pathway interruption familiar to every neurosurgeon. In the simplest terms, it is merely a matter of inserting a spinal needle of modest gauge into the spinal canal—a common maneuver to most neurosurgeons—then, under x-ray counselling, passing a special insulated stylet with tip designed for discrete coagulation through the hollow needle and introducing it into the anterolateral aspect of the cord. With properly developed skill, selective resection of the spinothalamic tract can be accomplished with reasonable consistency. In point of fact, this objective is attained in a gratifying percentage of cases by experienced operators. For the inexperienced, vexatious bobbing, lateral movement and twisting of an uncooperative spinal cord impose frustrating obstacles to successful lesion making, and a background in the rudiments of stereotaxis is essential. The procedure is not without hazards, and misplaced lesions by any technique at any level of skill may result. The list of complications includes all the possibilities we might expect from our knowledge of the functional anatomy of the cord plus a few newly observed adversities such as loss of the capacity for involuntary respiration during sleep, which is only beginning to be understood. Some of the initial problems are being resolved, as positional designation of the probe tip by impedance monitoring and more refined stimulation and evoked potential pick-up are providing physiological methods for more accurate lesion placement.

Uncontrollable suffering in patients with unalterably malignant conditions justifies an aggressive approach, especially in patients with advanced
debilitated states, if the method is simple and physically endurable. Percutaneous cordotomy, when applicable in these situations, is a welcome,
appropriate measure. The proper place of cordotomy in the expanding
catalogue of stereotaxic procedures will depend upon a sober analysis of
the long-term effects in patients treated by others for benign pain problems. Cordotomy has been discussed in greater depth in Chapter 5, in
which the explicit features of the posterior percutaneous method are
described.

OTHER AREAS OF STEREOTAXIC INTEREST

Categorization of stereotaxic endeavors as they relate to three major
operative designations is untenable beyond the format of this symposium.
Encephalotomy is a term generally used to imply supratentorial destruction of a brain area or pathway. Penetrating probes gliding beyond this
arbitrary level, particularly as they invade lower brain stem structures in
the posterior fossa, will produce results that certainly fall within the general category of encephalotomy, but characteristically will add distinctive
anatomical labelling. Mesencephalic tractotomy, imaginatively discussed
in Chapter 11, is an example of this deep invasion of the brain stem from
above (68). Intriguing speculation as to where the twain shall meet as
the downward penetration continues is engendered by the subject matter
of Chapter 9, describing a stereotaxic intrusion into the brain stem from
below for trigeminal tractotomy. Coincidental to the description of the
technical aspects of this lower approach, it is of interest that the most
remote lateral and central cerebellar targets are easily accessible in the
same positioning setup. The cerebellum is an area of relatively recent
stereotaxic concern (29), but as landmarks become more clearly defined,
greater attention will be attracted to the posterior fossa itself with its
complex sensory and motor associations that remain largely unfathomed
and, for the most part, stereotaxically virgin.

CONCLUSION

Stereotaxic surgery in human beings has progressed at a breathtaking
pace, with obvious accomplishments in difficult areas of pain and suffering. The rewards, though substantial, are dwarfed by realization of the
enormous potential application to a broadening spectrum of alterable
pathological entities involving the central nervous system. Knowledge ac-
quired by design or serendipity makes possible effective participation by
stereotaxic surgeons in favorable modification of pathological central

processes. Expansion of stereotaxic techniques and broader applications of the knowledge obtained poise stereotaxis on the threshold of new adventure. This promise is one of the exciting challenges of medicine today.

REFERENCES

1. ADAMS, J. E.; SEYMOUR, R. J.; EARLL, J. M.; TUCK, M.; SPARKS, L. L., and FORSHAM, P. H.: Transsphenoidal cryohypophysectomy in acromegaly: Clinical and endocrinological evaluation. *J Neurosurg,* 28:100, 1968.

2. ADEY, W. R.; RAND, R. W., and WALTER, R. D.: Depth stimulation and recording in thalamus and globus pallidus of patients with paralysis agitans. *J Nerv Ment Dis,* 129:417, 1959.

3. ALKSNE, J. F.; FINGERHUT, A., and RAND, R.: Magnetically controlled metallic thrombosis of intracranial aneurysms. *Surgery,* 60:212, 1966.

4. ANDY, O. J.: Globus pallidus coagulation technique. *Surg Forum,* 9:698, 1959.

5. ARONOW, S.: The use of radio-frequency power in making lesions in the brain. *J Neurosurg,* 17:431, 1960.

6. AUSTIN, G. M.; LEE, A. S. J., and GRANT, F. C.: A new type of locally applied stereotaxic instrument. *JAMA,* 161:147, 1956.

7. BALLANTINE, H. T., JR.; CASSIDY, W. L.; FLANAGAN, N. B., and MARINO, R., JR : Stereotaxic anterior cingulotomy for neuropsychiatric illness and intractable pain. *J Neurosurg,* 26:488, 1967.

8. BERTRAND, C., and MARTINEZ, N.: An apparatus and technique for surgery of dyskinesias. *Neurochirurgie,* 2:36, 1959.

9. BERTRAND, C.; MARTINEZ, N., and GAUTHIER, C.: Depth stimulation and recording in the course of stereotaxic surgery of the structures of the base of the brain. *Excerpta Medica,* 36:E55, 1961.

10. BRAVO, G., and COOPER, I. S.: Chemopallidectomy—two recent technical additions. *J Amer Geriat Soc,* 5:651, 1957.

11. BRAVO, G. J., and COOPER, I. S.: A clinical and radiological correlation of the lesions produced by chemopallidectomy and thalamectomy. *J Neurol Neurosurg Psychiat,* 22:1, 1959.

12. BRAZIER, M. A. B.; KJELLBERG, R. N.; SWEET, W. H., and BARLOW, J. S.: Electrographic recording and correlation analysis from deep structures within the human brain. In Ramey, E. R., and O'Doherty, D. S. (Eds.): *Electrical Studies on the Unanesthetized Brain.* New York, Hoeber, 1960, pp. 311-328.

13. CONWAY, L. W.; O'FOGHLUDHA, F. T., and COLLINS, W. F.: Stereotaxic treatment of acromegaly. *J Neurol Neurosurg Psychiat,* 32:48, 1969.

14. COOPER, I. S.: Intracerebral injection of procaine into the globus pallidus in hyperkinetic disorders. *Science,* 119:417, 1954.

15. COOPER, I. S.: Clinical results and follow-up studies in a personal series of 300 operations for parkinsonism. *J Amer Geriat Soc,* 4:1171, 1956.

16. COOPER, I. S.: The neurosurgical alleviation of parkinsonism. Springfield, Thomas, 1956.

17. CRANDALL, P. H.; WALTER, R. D., and RAND, R. W.: Clinical applications of studies on stereotactically implanted electrodes in temporal lobe epilepsy. *J Neurosurg,* 20:827, 1963.

18. DELGADO, J. M. R.: Functional exploration of the brain with stereotaxic techniques. *J Neurosurg,* 15:269, 1958.

19. DONALDSON, A. A.: Surgical management of the dyskinesias. *J Neurol Neurosurg Psychiat,* 23:348, 1960.
20. FAGER, C. A.: Technique of stereotactic surgery. *Surg Clin N Amer,* 40:575, 1960.
21. FEINSTEIN, B.; ALBERTS, W. W.; WRIGHT, E. W., JR., and LEVIN, G.: A stereotaxic technique in man allowing multiple spatial and temporal approaches to intracranial targets. *J Neurosurg,* 17:708, 1960.
22. FOLTZ, E. L., and WHITE, L. E., JR.: Pain "relief" by frontal cingulumotomy. *J Neurosurg,* 19:89, 1962.
23. GASS, H. H.: Personal Communication.
24. GILLINGHAM, F. J.; WATSON, W. S.; DONALDSON, A. A., and NAUGHTON, J. A. L.: The surgical treatment of parkinsonism. *Brit Med J,* 2:1395, 1960.
25. GROS, C.; ROILGEN, A., and VLAHOVITCH, B.: Pallidotomy and thalamotomy in Parkinson's disease. *J Neurol Neurosurg Psychiat,* 23:350, 1960.
26. GUIOT, G.: Le traitement des syndromes parkinsoniens par la destruction du pallidum interne. *Neurochirurgie,* 1:94, 1958.
27. HARDY, J., and BERTRAND, C.: Electrophysiological exploration of sub-cortical structure with microelectrode during stereotaxic surgery. (See Spiegel and Wycis, Part I, pp. 201, No. 461, 1966.
28. HASSLER, R.; RIECHERT, T.; MUDINGER, F.; UNBACK, W., and GANGELBERGER, J. A.: Physiological observations in stereotaxic operations in extrapyramidal motor disturbances. *Brain,* 83:337, 1960.
29. HEIMBURGER, R. F., and WHITLOCK, C. C.: Stereotaxic destruction of the human dentate nucleus. (See Spiegel and Wycis, Part I, pp. 346, No. 461, 1966).
30. HEIMBURGER, R. F.; WHITLOCK, C. C., and KOLSBECK, J. E.: Stereotaxic amygdalotomy for epilepsy with aggressive behavior. *JAMA,* 198:741, 1966.
31. HODGES, P. C., and GARCIA-BENGOCHEA, F.: Precise alignment of x-ray beams for stereotaxic surgery. *Amer J Roentgen,* 105:260, 1969.
32. HORSLEY, V., and CLARKE, R. H.: The structure and functions of cerebellum examined by a new method. *Brain,* 31:45, 1908.
33. JASPER, H. H.: Recording from microelectrodes in stereotactic surgery for Parkinson's disease. *J Neurosurg,* 24:219, 1966.
34. KJELLBERG, R. N., and SWEET, W. H.: Stereotactic surgery for involuntary movements. (See von Bogaert and Radermecker, pp. 56, No. 530, 1957.)
35. KRAYENBUHL, H.: Discussion of stereotaxic coagulation. *Confin Neurol,* 22:314, 1962.
36. LAITINEN, L.; JOHANSSON, G. G., and SIPPONEN, P.: Impedance and phase angle as a locating method in human stereotaxic surgery. *J Neurosurg,* 25:628, 1966.
37. LE BEAU, J.; DONDEY, M., and ALBE-FESSARD, D.: Determination de la fonction de certaines structures cerebrales profondes par refroidissement localise et reversible. *Rev Neurol (Paris),* 107:485, 1962.
38. LEKSELL, L.: A stereotaxic apparatus for intracerebral surgery. *Acta Chir Scand,* 99:229, 1949.
39. LIN, T. H., and COOPER, I. S.: Results of chemopallidectomy and chemothalamectomy. A study of one hundred cases of parkinsonism and ages over sixty. *Arch Neurol (Chicago),* 2:188, 1960.
40. MARK, V. H.; ERVIN, F. R., and HACKETT, T. P.: Clinical aspects of stereotactic thalamotomy in the human. Part I. The treatment of chronic severe pain. *Arch Neurol (Chicago),* 3:351, 1960.
41. MARK, V. H., and HACKETT, T. P.: Surgical aspects of thalamotomy in the human. *Trans Amer Neurol Ass,* 84:92, 1959.

42. MARKHAM, C. H., and RAND, R. W.: Stereotactic surgery in Parkinson's disease. *Arch Neurol (Chicago)*, 8:621, 1963.
43. MASON, M. S.: Personal Communication.
44. McKINNEY, W. W. (Reference to be inserted in galley proof.)
45. MEYERS, R.; FRY, W. J.; FRY, F. J.; DREYER, L. L.; SCHULTZ, D. F., and NOYES, R. F.: Early experiences with ultrasonic irradiation of the pallidofugal and nigral complexes in hyperkinetic and hypertonic disorders. *J Neurosurg*, 16:32, 1959.
46. MULLAN, S.; RAIMONDI, A. J.; DOBBEN, G.; VAILATI, C., and HEKMATPANAH, J.: Electrically induced thrombosis in intracranial aneurysms. *J Neurosurg*, 22:539, 1965.
47. MULLAN, S.; VAILATI, G.; KARASICK, J., and MAILIS, M.: Thalamic lesions for the control of epilepsy. A study of nine cases. *Arch Neurol (Chicago)*, 16:277, 1967.
48. MUNDINGER, F., and RIECHERT, T.: Stereotaxic brain operations for the treatment of extrapyramidal movement disorders (parkinsonism and hyperkinesias) and their results. *Fortschr Neurol Psychiat*, 31:1 and 69, 1963.
49. NARABAYASHI, H., and OKUMA, T.: Procaine oil block of the globus pallidus for the treatment of rigidity and tremor of parkinsonism. *Proc Japan Acad*, 29:310, 1953.
50. NASHOLD, B. S., JR., and WILSON, W. P.: Central pain. Observation in man with chronic implanted electrodes in the midbrain tegmentum. (See Spiegel and Wycis, Part II, pp. 30, No. 462, 1966.)
51. OBRADOR, S., and DIERSSEN, G.: Personal experience in the treatment of parkinsonian symptoms with subcortical operations. (See van Bogaert and Radermecker, pp. 119, No. 530, 1957.)
52. RAND, R. W.; HEUSER, G.; DASHE, A.; ADAMS, D., and ROTH, N.: Stereotaxic transsphenoidal biopsy and cryosurgery of pituitary tumors. *Amer J Roentgen*, 105:260, 1969.
53. RAND, R. W.: A stereotaxic instrument for pallidothalamectomy in Parkinson's disease. *J Neurosurg*, 18, 258, 1961.
54. RIECHERT, T.: Long term follow-up of results of stereotaxic treatment in extrapyramidal disorders. *Confin Neurol*, 22:356, 1962.
55. Riechert, T., and Mundinger, F.: Stereotaxic instruments. (See Schaltenbrand and Bailey, pp. 439, No. 439, 1959.)
56. SACHS, E.: On the structure and functional relations of the optic thalamus. *Brain*, 32:95, 1909.
57. SACHS, E., and FINCHER, E. F., JR.: Anatomical and physiological observations on lesions in the cerebellar nuclei in Macacus rhesus. *Brain*, 50:350, 1927.
58. SPIEGEL, E. A.; WYCIS, H. T., and FREED, H.: Stereoencephalotomy. Thalamotomy and related procedures. *JAMA*, 148:446, 1952.
59. SPIEGEL, E. A.; WYCIS, H. T.; MARKS, M., and LEE, A. J.: Stereotaxic apparatus for operations on the human brain. *Science*, 106:349, 1947.
60. SWEET, W. H.; MARK, V. H., and HAMLIN, H.: Radiofrequency lesions in central nervous system of man and cat: including case reports of eight bulbar pain-tract interruptions. *J Neurosurg*, 17:213, 1960.
61. TAARNHOJ, J.; ARNOIS, D. C., and DONAHUE, L. A.: Chemopallidectomy as a treatment for Parkinson's disease. Evaluation of results in 118 patients. *J Neurosurg*, 17:459, 1960.
62. TALAIRACH, J.: Les explorations radiologiques stereotaxiques. *Rev Neurol (Paris)*, 90:556, 1954.
63. TALAIRACH, J.; DAVID, M., and TOURNOUX, P.: L'exploration chirurgicale stereotaxique

du lobe temporal dans l'epilepsie temporal. *Reperage anatomique stereotaxique et technique chirurgicale*. Paris, Masson & Cie, 1958.

64. TODD, E. M.: *Manual of Stereotaxic Procedures*. Privately published by Mechanical Developments Company, South Gate, California, 1967.

65. TODD, E. M., and CRUE, B. L., JR.: An image enlargement scale for stereotactic surgery. *Amer J Roentgen*, 105:270, 1969.

66. TODD, E. M.; SHELDON, C. H.; PUDENZ, R. H., and CRUE, B. L., JR.: Surgical management of dyskinesia. *Amer J Surg*, 102:265, 1961.

67. UMBACH, W.: Cortical responses to subcortical stimulation of the diffuse projecting system in 622 stereotaxic operations in man. *Excerpta Medica*, 37:76, 1962.

68. WARD, A. A., JR.: Trends in the application of stereotaxy to the brain stem. *Clin Neurosurg*, 6:233, 1959.

69. WYCIS, H. T., and SPIEGEL, E. A.: Thalamotomy and mesencephalothalamotomy: neurosurgical aspects (including treatment of pain). *New York J Med*, 49:2275, 1949.

70. WYCIS, H. T., and SPIEGEL, E. A.: Long-range results in the treatment of intractable pain by stereotaxic midbrain surgery. *J Neurosurg*, 19:101, 1962.

71. YOSHIDA, M.; YANAGISAWA, N.; SHIMAZU, H.; GIVRE, A., and NARABAYASHI, H.: Physiological identification of the thalamic nucleus. *Arch Neurol (Chicago)*, 11:435, 1964.

72. ZERVAS, N. T., and GORDY, P. D.: Radiofrequency hypophysectomy for metastatic breast and prostatic carcinoma. *Surg Clin N Amer*, 47: 1279, 1967.

Chapter 11

CENTRAL PAIN AND THE IRRITABLE MIDBRAIN

BLAINE S. NASHOLD, JR. AND WILLIAM P. WILSON

> Of course, this is speculative. I am not aware that anyone pretends to know the seat or the pathology of cases of "genuine epilepsy." I think that these are "lowest level fits." These are fits produced by excessive discharges beginning in parts of the lowest level, a level which is common to the cerebral and the cerebellar systems. I suppose that most of them are owing to excessive discharges beginning in centres of the bulbar and pontal regions of the level, hence I sometimes use the term "ponto-bulbar fits." (10)
>
> HUGHLINGS JACKSON, 1890

TO the physician, pain of central origin represents a complexity of symptoms that are puzzling and difficult to treat. To a patient, suffering from pain, the experience may be so devastating as to threaten his mental and physical existence. To the neurophysiologist, a study of central pain phenomena in man may offer an opportunity to test the current theories on the neural mechanisms of pain. Total relief from central pain by the application of current therapies still eludes us. The neurosurgeon's interest in central pain has increased of late for several reasons. One has been the introduction of stereotaxic neurosurgical techniques that allow the surgeon to interrupt pain pathways at certain levels in the CNS either by percutaneous or transcerebral routes (16, 17, 25, 28). Secondly, the neurosurgeon has become keenly aware that a therapeutic lesion that interrupts pain pathways may predispose his patient to the terrible risk of central pain. The clinical facts associated with the syndromes of central pain are well documented in the literature, but there still exists a lack of understanding of its pathophysiology.

Recently, Cassinari and Pagni (3) have reviewed and summarized the clinical and theoretical aspects associated with the causes of central pain and they conclude that central pain is a central irritative phenomenon. They state: "A group of theories that would seem to be unassailable are those based on irritation. No one can rule out the possibility that fibers and cells at lesion level undergo an irritative process and that this is one of the fundamental factors in the genesis of central pain."

In 1965, Nashold and Wilson (17) studied and reported in detail a woman with central pain in whom depth electrodes were chronically implanted in her thalamus and midbrain. She suffered from severe paroxysms of right facial pain which occurred a year after a serious subarachnoid hemorrhage. Spontaneous and evoked epileptic discharges were recorded from the midbrain in association with her facial pain. Since then, further observations have been carried out in a group of fifteen persons with central pain due to spontaneous lesions at various sites in the CNS. Electrodes were implanted into the thalamic and dorsal mesencephalon for stimulation and later, at a second operation, HF lesions were made (18, 19). Three patients have exhibited either electrographic or clinical manifestation of hyperirritability of the dorsal midbrain and adjacent thalamus. The observations reported in this paper give further support to the idea that central pain in certain patients may be due to an irritable midbrain.

CASE REPORTS

Case 1 (V. H.)

This 46-year-old female sustained a subarachnoid hemorrhage in 1961 that left her with a left hemiplegia, aphasia, hemianalgesia and homonymous hemianopsia. Angiography did not reveal the source of the bleeding, but she did recover and a year later began to suffer from severe paroxysms of right facial pain. The pain involved the entire right half of the face, but was more severe in the region of the cheek. During the attacks of pain her face would become red, with a blush spreading over the right side of her neck and shoulder. The pain was of two types; one a sudden severe lancinating pain which made her cry out. She would press her hand to the cheek as if its pressure gave her some relief. This pain was paroxysmal and lasted for many seconds. The severest pains were often followed by a generalized convulsive seizure. The seizures began after a left frontal lobotomy which failed to relieve the pain. The seizures occurred without pain and were difficult to control with medication. The seizures were controlled, however, after the midbrain lesion was made which relieved the pain. The second type was a dull, aching pain in the region of the cheek. She was aware of this most of the time, but its intensity was lessened by rest and analgesics. Loud noises and emotional upsets increased the intensity of both types of the pain. Unsuccessful attempts had been made to relieve the pain by injections of local analgesics or alcohol into the branches of the trigeminal nerves in the area of pain. A unilateral left frontal lobotomy was also unsuccessful in relieving the pain.

Clinical examination (three years after the episode of subarachnoid hemorrhage and hemiplegia): She was 49 years old, alert and cooperative despite an expressive aphasia. She could answer with "yes" or "no," and seemed to comprehend spoken and written words well. She had been an accomplished musician and could still sing a few lines from her favorite songs. Examination of the cranial nerves revealed a right central facial paresis. The visual acuity was normal, but examinations of the visual fields revealed a right incongruous homonymous hemianopsia. There was a right spastic hemiplegia with hyperactive deep tendon reflexes and an extensor toe response to plantar stimulation. A hemianalgesia was noted over the right half of her body with a decrease in the appreciation of pinprick, which was also unpleasant to her. Thermal sensation was reduced over the entire right half of the body, but hot or cold objects were also unpleasant. Light touch was poorly localized, while position sense was partially preserved in the toes.

Many paroxysms of the "thalamic" pain were observed. The patient seemed to have a brief one-to-two-second warning and then would cry out "oh, oh, oh!" She would then put her left hand to the right cheek and exert pressure. A grimace would distort her face and she would roll her eyes as if in agony. The skin over the face and right side of the neck and shoulder would turn red and she would sweat profusely. The painful attacks lasted many seconds and then would subside, leaving a residual aching in the cheek. There were no trigger areas on the face or in the mouth.

It was decided to make a lesion in the region of the left quinto-thalamic tract at the level of the midbrain. Because electrical stimulation and EEG recordings from the brain at the time of a stereotaxic operation is less than satisfactory, we decided to implant a series of multiple contact depth electrodes in the brain and brain stem and make a systematic study of the patient's clinical state under the best possible circumstances, with the hope of improving the site of the therapeutic lesion.

A group of six depth electrodes were implanted in the left brain. These electrodes have been described elsewhere (17) in detail but consisted of six contacts for recording and stimulation space either at 5 or 10 mm. Bipolar EEG recordings were made and stimulation was carried out between adjacent contacts of the same electrode. The designation of contacts in the EEG recordings were from the most caudal contact (one) to rostral (six).

Two electrodes were placed over the cortical surface of the frontal and parietal regions (Fig. 11-1) and the third was inserted into the white matter between the two cortical electrodes. Three electrodes were implanted stereotaxically into the left sensory thalamus and midbrain. The thalamus electrode was oriented to the region of the posterolateral thalamus, the midbrain electrodes were placed in the dorsal tegmentum and ventral tegmentum in the region of the medial lemniscus and lateral bor-

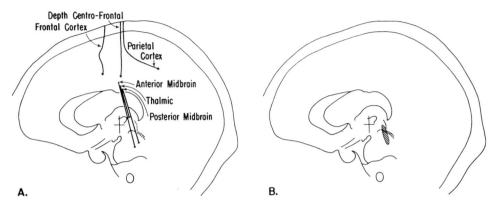

Figure 11-1. Patient 1 (V. H.) A. Location of implanted chronic left cortical, thalamic and brain stem electrodes. Patient's right facial pain produced from tip (contacts 1-2, 10 mm separation) of posterior (dorsal) brain stem electrode. Spontaneous and evoked epileptic activity recorded from same region. B. Location of HF Lesions which relieved pain.

der of the red nucleus. The electrodes were left *in situ* for sixteen days for EEG recordings and stimulation. The patient was alert during these procedures.

A Grass stimulator S4 with isolation unit was used. Unidirectional pulses were delivered at 0.1 to 1.0 msec. duration with variation in voltage and rate. The contact resistance ranged from 40 to 60,000 ohms with current flow measured between 2 to 4 ma.

RESULTS OF ELECTROGRAPHIC RECORDINGS

Preoperative and postoperative scalp EEG's: The resting rhythms from the right cerebral hemisphere were normal. In the parieto-occipital region there was an alpha rhythm of 50 to 70μv mixed with minimal beta rhythms which also occurred in the temporal region. Beta activity was the predominant rhythm in the anterior portion of the brain. The findings were similar in the preoperative and postoperative records. Hyperventilation did not alter the preoperative record.

The rhythms from the left hemisphere were abnormal. Slow activity in the delta (1-3 cps) and theta (4-7 cps) frequency range occurred in the F3-C3 and C3-P3 electrode combinations. More delta than theta activity was noted in the region of the temporal lobe. Epileptic discharges consisting of sharp waves and slow spikes were observed in the left frontotemporal regions, but were most numerous in the temporal region. Definite improvement occurred in the postoperative record, with decreased slowing of activity and fewer epileptic discharges.

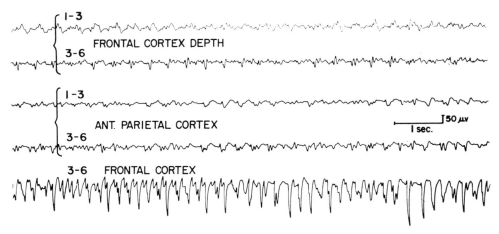

Figure 11-2. Spontaneous epileptic spikes in the left frontal cortex (result of frontal lobotomy which failed to relieve facial pain) associated with right-sided focal motor seizures. Patient did not complain of pain and remained conscious.

Left frontal cortical electrode: The electrical activity consisted of spikes occurring at intervals of 3 to 4 seconds, or as often as 2 to 3 per second. The voltage varied and the spikes did not occur in bursts. A spontaneous electrographic seizure was recorded from the left frontal lobe (Fig. 11-2). Low voltage beta and alpha rhythms were also noted with the alpha rhythm occurring at 8 cps.

Electrical stimulation of the left frontal cortex produced a focal motor seizure with myoclonic rhythmic movements of the face, tongue and arm. Stimuli used were at 10, 60, 100 and 300 cps from 10 to 50 volts with pulse durations of 1 msec.

Anterior parietal lobe cortical electrode: The electrical activity from the parietal cortex consisted of multiple spikes of about 100 μv in amplitude that occurred singly or as bursts of several spikes at 6 per second. Beta rhythms were mixed with the spike activity, with bursts every 1 to 3 seconds (Fig. 11-3).

Electrical stimulation of the parietal cortex at frequencies of 10, 60, 100 and 300/sec. at voltages ranging from 5 to 75 volts failed to alter the electrical activity of the brain. There were no subjective responses.

Left fronto-parietal white matter depth electrode: The EEG activity was low voltage with minimal beta activity and slow theta.

Electrical stimulation frequencies of 10, 60, 100 and 300 cps with 5 to 15 volts and pulses of 0.1 and 1 msec duration failed to elicit electrographic or subjective responses.

Left thalamic depth electrode: The spontaneous activity in the thala-

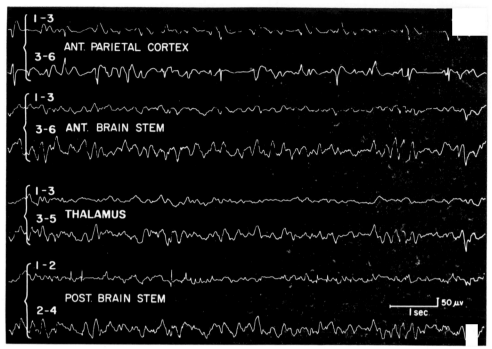

Figure 11-3. Epileptic activity from left anterior parietal cortex and independent epileptic spike activity recorded from left dorsal brain tegmentum. The electrical activity in the other two electrodes is comprised mostly of slow waves.

mic electrode was negligible in the more caudal electrode contacts, 1, 2 and 3. There were low voltage rhythms of all frequencies in the more rostral electrode contacts, 4, 5 and 6. There were alpha, beta and theta rhythms of moderate voltage. Epileptic discharges were not seen.

Stimulation of all points of this electrode at frequencies of 5, 10, 60, 100 and 300 cps at 15 volts with pulse durations of 0.1 and 1 msec failed to elicit abnormal discharge or behavioral activity.

Left ventral (anterior) midbrain depth electrode: The EEG rhythms were high voltage predominated by theta activity. These rhythms were recorded from the rostral recording contacts of this electrode. Low voltage beta activity mixed with theta rhythms was recorded from this electrode. No epileptic discharge was noted. Low voltage beta and theta activity was observed at the caudal tip of electrode points 1, 2 and 3, but there was no epileptic discharge.

Electrical stimulation at frequencies of 10, 60, 100 and 300 cps with 5, 10, and 15 volts at durations of 0.1 and 1.0 msec did not alter the electrical activity.

Left dorsal (posterior) midbrain depth electrode: Caudal contacts 1

and 2 of this electrode were in the left dorsal tegmentum with contacts 1 and 2 approximately 1 to 3 mm from the midline. The distance
between the electrode points was 10 mm. When spontaneous paroxysms
of right facial pain occurred, there appeared in the tegmentum spike
activity grouped in trains lasting for the duration of the pain (Fig. 11-4).
The activity from this region consisted of small low voltage fast spikes of
less than 5 msec duration in the intervals between the pain. When the
spontaneous spike activity occurred in the left dorsal tegmentum, there

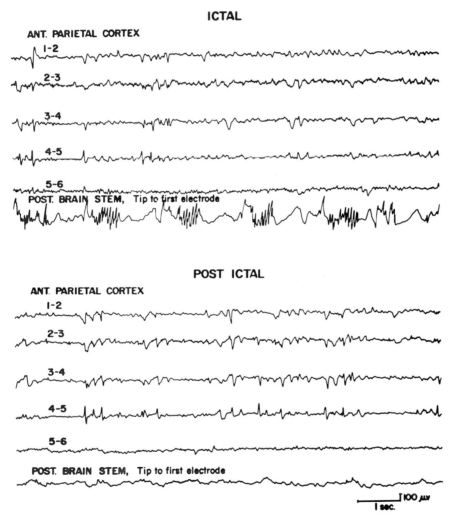

Figure 11-4. *Ictal* epileptic activity recorded from left dorsal brain stem tegmentum at
most caudal contacts at level of colliculus. Patient experiences right facial pain during
period of epileptic activity. Note absence of seizure paroxysms in the left parietal cortex.
Postictal tracing after facial pain ceased shows flattening of EEG.

was no alteration of the EEG from the nearby electrode in the left ventral tegmentum or from the cortical or deep frontal electrodes. The second type of pain, which was dull and aching in nature, was associated with spikes of small voltage from the dorsal tegmental region.

Bipolar electrical stimulation of the left dorsal tegmentum reproduced severe paroxysms of right facial pains and initiated the spike activity, which continued beyond the end of the stimulation (Figs. 11-5, 11-6). When the pain had ceased, the spike activity stopped. The most intense pain followed stimulation, using unidirectional square waves of 1 msec duration at frequencies of 100 to 300 cps with 10 to 15 volts. She dreaded the effects of stimulation as she had dreaded her spontaneous facial pains. Unpleasant sensations of the right face were also evoked from stimulation in the region of the left medial lemniscus. Stimulation of the thalamic electrode resulted in unpleasant sensations but no pain. The intensity of the pain seemed to be augmented by stimulation if there was an increased awareness or anxiety as she anticipated the pain. The dull pains in the right face waxed and waned in concert with the low voltage spikes noted in the EEG recordings from the left mesencephalon.

A spontaneous severe paroxysm of facial pain might end with a generalized motor seizure. It was not possible to produce this sequence of

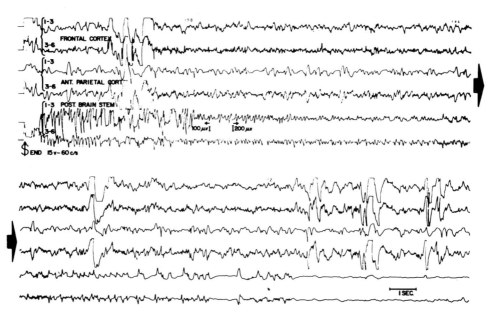

Figure 11-5. Epileptic activity recorded from left dorsal midbrain tegmentum following electrical stimulation which also reproduced right facial pain that continued beyond end of stimulation. Facial pain stopped when epileptic discharges stopped and EEG became flat.

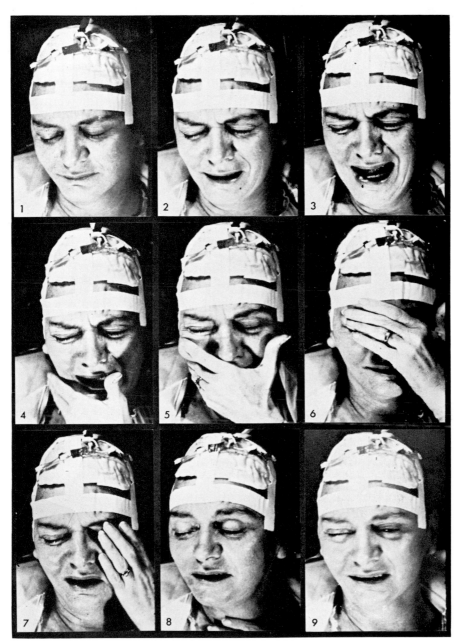

Figure 11-6. Response of the patient associated with electrical stimulation of left dorsal mesencephalic tegmentum electrode in the same region where the spontaneous epileptic discharges were recorded when patient experienced spontaneous right facial pain without stimulation. Parameters of stimulation were 100 Hz, 0.1 msec duration pulse, 5 volts, 2 seconds. Frame No. 1—before stimulation. Frame No. 2—onset of stimulus. Frame No. 3 to 5—painful right facial sensation continues after stimulus off. Patient crying "oh, oh, oh" with the onset of irregular breathing, blush occurring over right side of face and shoulder. Frames 6 to 9—recovery, no vocalization, autonomic signs of sweating and blushing continue, dull aching sensation in face.

103

events by brain stem stimulation, although convulsive adversive seizures did occur from stimulation of the cerebral cortex of the frontal lobe. The patient first put her hand to her cheek and this was followed by clonic jerks of all extremities and deviation of her eyes to the contralateral side. After the convulsive seizures, the patient indicated that she had some intensification of the pain in the face which lasted long after the seizures had stopped.

Case 2 (P. B.)

This 61-year-old male had central pain for 38 years involving the right face, arm and chest due to a traumatic parietal and stereotaxic midbrain lesion.

In 1928, he fell 25 feet into an elevator shaft and sustained a broken wrist. There was no evidence of brain injury then, but three weeks later he had a series of generalized epileptic seizures and headaches. He was examined at Johns Hopkins Hospital by Dr. Walter Dandy who noted bilateral papilledema. At operation Dandy described a cystic lesion of the left parieto-occipital region, and an occipital lobectomy was done. The exact pathologic nature of the lesion was never clear, but tumor and/or trauma were considered. The man recovered except for a visual field defect. He continued to have occasional seizures that were controlled with anticonvulsants.

In 1953, he began to complain of severe pain in the right arm. Spiegel and Wycis (25) examined him and believed the pain to be of central origin; they performed a left stereotaxic midbrain lesion. Postoperatively, he developed a mild hemiparesis with temporary relief of the pain. As time went on, however, the pain intensified and spread to involve his face, chest and arm. In 1969, the senior author examined him at Duke Hospital, and at the time he was complaining bitterly of pain in the right face, chest and arm. His wife said he had become desperate because of the pain, suffering bouts of depression and threatening suicide. The examination revealed an alert but depressed man complaining of pain. He held his glove-covered right hand in a protective manner at his side. There was a mild right spastic hemiparesis plus a central facial paresis, but he could walk using a cane. The tendon reflexes were hyperactive on the right side. There was a mild to moderate analgesia and thermal anesthesia in the right arm and hand. The skin of his right face, arm and chest was hyperalgesic. Spontaneous pains could be evoked by touch, cold or pulling the hairs on the right arm.

I thought that his original pain had developed because of a traumatic lesion involving the left parietal lobe. Later, the pain was intensified by the stereotaxic midbrain lesion. The patient stated that the hyperalgesia

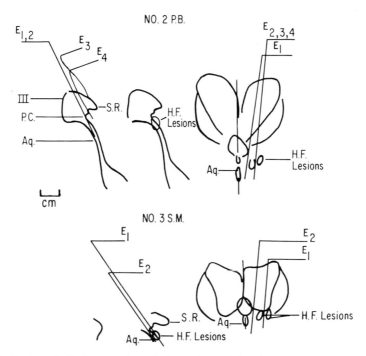

Figure 11-7. *Patient 2 (P. B.)* Tracing of electrode position from x ray.
E 1 medial midbrain electrode 3-6 mm from midline. EEG recording contacts separated 5 mm.
E 2 lateral midbrain electrode 8-10 mm from midline. Electrode lateral and parallel to E 1. EEG recording contacts separated 2 mm.
E 3 pulvinar electrode. EEG recording contacts separated 5 mm.
E 4 pretectal electrode. EEG recording contacts separated 5 mm.
HF lesions—two at rostral level of midbrain lateral and parallel to aqueduct, ventral to colliculus.
Each lesion produced at 70° C/30 sec.

Patient 3 (S. M.)
E 1 lateral midbrain electrode 9-10 mm from midline. EEG recording contacts separated 2 mm.
E 2 medial midbrain electrode 3-6.5 mm from midline. EEG recording contacts separated 2 mm.
HF lesions—two in rostral midbrain produced at 70-72° C/30 sec.

> III—posterior third ventricle.
> P.C.—posterior commissure.
> Aq.—Sylvian aqueduct.
> S.R.—Suprapineal recess.

was recent, and although his original spontaneous pain was unchanged since the parietal injury, it had now spread to involve a larger area of the body (arm-chest).

In September of 1966 (38 years after the left parietal lesion and 7 years following left mesencephalic lesion), a series of four depth electrodes was implanted into the left thalamus and midbrain in the region of the previous stereotaxic surgery (Fig. 11-7).

Two electrodes were introduced into the left mesencephalon lateral to the aqueduct and beneath the collicular plate. The medial electrode with its lowest contacts was estimated to be at 3 to 4 mm from the aqueduct in the mesial mesencephalon. The rostral contacts of this electrode were in the mesial thalamic region (md and parafascicularis, 5 to 6 mm from 3rd ventricle). The electrode in the dorsolateral midbrain was estimated to be 8.5 to 10 mm from the midaqueduct (spinothalamic and quinto-thalamic tract), with its rostral contacts in the centre median nucleus of the thalamus. The other two electrodes were oriented more dorsolaterally (8 to 9 mm and 12 to 14 mm from mid-third ventricle), in the pretectal and pulvinar regions.

STIMULATION RESULTS

Mesial Midbrain: Unpleasant sensations were produced. They were characterized by the patient as a "frightening feeling." These feelings occurred during high frequency stimulation, which intensified the spontaneous pain in the right arm. Contralateral and ipsilateral piloerection (arm and chest), sighing respirations, decreased GSR (arm), oscillations of the eyes and closure of the eyelids occurred with these electrical stimulations.

Dorsolateral Midbrain: Burning pains were reproduced in the right face, arm, chest and trunk, but none in the abdomen or leg. Deep respirations occurred during the stimulation, but no change occurred in the EKG, cardiac rate or plethysmographic recording. Contralateral piloerection (arm-chest) occurred which was sustained poststimulation. The pain in the arm also persisted in the poststimulation period from 15 to 30 seconds.

Thalamic pretectal: The sensations were contralateral, localized mainly in the right face and abdomen, and described only vaguely. The patient felt "dizziness," "numbness" or "tingling," but no pain was elicited from the pulvinar. He experienced sensations referred to the stomach and abdominal cavity during stimulation of the midline thalamic regions. Epileptic after-discharges were recorded from the pretectal region during and after stimulation, but no behavioral changes occurred (Fig. 11-8).

Four HF lesions were made in the left dorsolateral mesencephalon in

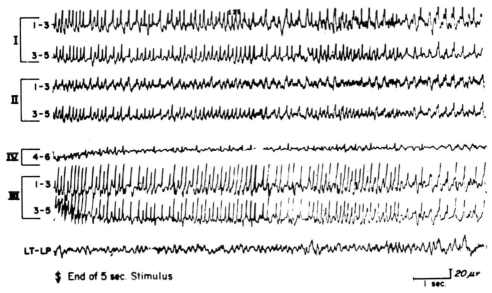

$ End of 5 sec. Stimulus   20 μv
                                            1 sec.

Figure 11-8. *Patient 2 (P. B.)* After-discharge recorded from left dorsal tegmentum. Electrode positions 1 (see Fig. 11-7). Contacts 1-3 inferior to superior colliculus, 3-5 pretectum and central median.
E II contacts 1-3 mesencephalic tegmentum, 3-5 lateral tegmentum.
E IV contacts 4-6 pulvinar.
E III contacts 1-3 pulvinar, 3-5 medial dorsal thalamus.
Parameters of stimulation: 60 Hz, 1 msec duration, 10 volts, 5 seconds.

the region in which stimulation reproduced the burning pain referred to the right arm, face and chest. After the operation, the degree of analgesia was increased over the face, arm and chest. The burning pain and hyperanalgesia were relieved. He still complained of an undefined discomfort in his hand. He exhibited an immediate loss of upward gaze, nystagmus retractorius, loss of convergence, and miosis. The patient was improved and remained so for the next two years, although he did suffer from bouts of depression. He died suddenly from an acute subdural hemorrhage, and a preliminary examination of his brain revealed an atrophic lesion in the left parietal lobe. Studies are underway on the thalamus and midbrain.

CONCLUSION

This patient had an extremely complex history with two separate pathologic insults to the CNS, the first involving the parieto-occipital cortex and the second as the result of the first stereotaxic lesion in the dorsolateral mesencephalon. The intensity of his pain was initially reduced, only to be followed later by an intensification of the pain over a

larger area of the body. It is likely that after the first stereotaxic operation, he suffered from a postmesencephalic dysesthesia imposed on his
original pain response. A zone of hyperirritability may have developed
adjacent to the first stereotaxic lesion in the dorsal midbrain, resulting
in the hyperalgesia. Stimulation of the dorsal midbrain in or near the
first stereotaxic lesion activated irritable neural tissue, reproducing the
spontaneous burning pain. The persistence of the pain poststimulation
may have resulted from an after-discharge effect, although at the time
no electrographic epileptic activity was recorded. Epileptic after-discharges were recorded from the pretectal-thalamic junction zone, rostral
to the lesion, following local stimulation of this area, but no behavioral
or sensory change was noted.

Case 3 (S. M.)

In December of 1965, this 66-year-old female underwent a hemor-
rhoidectomy. Twenty-four hours postoperatively she lapsed into a coma
and developed a right hemiparesis. A left brachial and a right carotid
angiogram were negative. Spinal fluid examination was normal. She recovered gradually but was confused and exhibited a right hemiparesis
and aphasia. Four weeks later, tremor of the head and right arm were
observed. She tended to perseverate when she spoke. At this time she
began to complain of unpleasant burning or freezing sensations involving
the right side of her body. During this time she was confused and depressed.

She was examined at Duke in October 1966, and the neurological examination revealed a right-handed woman with speech perseveration. Her
past memory was fair, but her recent memory poor.

The cranial nerve examination showed normal ocular movements and
light reflexes. The visual fields were normal. Voluntary facial movements
were normal except for an involuntary right facial tic. These involuntary
twitchings were centered around the mouth and tongue. There was a
slight motor weakness of the right hand and leg. Passive motion of the
right arm and leg was associated with a mild increase in muscle tone
and cogging. Voluntary right arm movements were jerky and irregular,
with a superimposed intention tremor. She had poor fine finger coordination on the right hand, and the extended fingers assumed a posture of
hyperextension at the metacarpal phalangeal joints. The tendon reflexes
were hypertonic on the right, but no Hoffman or Babinski signs were
present. Her gait was unusual because she was unbalanced when she
walked with a tendency to keep the right leg in rigid extension. It was not
a typical hemiplegic gait. She described the pain as "burning" or a "block
of ice," but there was no distortion of her body image. The corneal and

nasal tickle reactions were normal. Light touch was normal. Vibration and position sense were normal. On some occasions, a light touch was slightly more sensitive over the right cheek, but the right arm was hyperalgesic to pinprick. Her response to a pinprick on the arm was always delayed for a few seconds but then she would withdraw the arm, grimace and describe an unpleasant feeling. She could not distinguish between hot or cold in the arm, but would withdraw it complaining of some discomfort with thermal application. A moderate analgesia was present on her face and arm.

SPECIAL EXAMINATIONS

The brain scan, pneumoencephalogram, EEG and audiograms were normal.

The summary of the psychological testing revealed a bright normal range of intelligence when dealing with previously learned and well-practiced verbal material. There was marked impairment of new verbal and perceptual learning tasks. Both the quantitative and qualitative features of her performance suggested a strong organic impairment of her present intellectual functioning.

CLINICAL COURSE

In November 1966, two chronic electrodes were inserted into the left dorsal mesencephalon (Fig. 7). The medial electrode was oriented 3 to 6.5 mm from the midline and parallel to the sylvian aqueduct beneath the colliculus. It was estimated that the electrode contacts were in mesial dorsal mesencephalon beneath the colliculus and extended rostrally into the parabigeminal region dorsal to the red nucleus. A second electrode was oriented more laterally at 9 to 10 mm, extending from the dorsolateral tegmentum in the region of the lateral spinothalamic tract with the rostral contacts in the medial pulvinar. Isolated epileptic spikes were recorded from the rostral pulvinar, but they were not related to her spontaneous pain nor could pain be elicited from the pulvinar region.

Stimulation of the caudal contacts in the mesial midbrain on the left resulted in unpleasant sensations described as "fearful" and "frightening." She localized this feeling to the center of her face. Stimulation of the more lateral midbrain electrode contacts (6.5 mm) resulted in a burning and painful sensation referred to the lateral aspects of the face, neck and chest. Activation of the facial pain by stimulation in lateral midbrain was also associated with activation of the facial tic. High frequency stimulation (120 to 300 Hz, 5 volts, 1 msec) was followed by a right-sided clonic facial spasm (similar to her spontaneous tic) in addition to a rhythmical twitching of the eyelids and a rhythmically contralateral conjugate upward deviation of the eyes. This complex facio-ocular seizure persisted beyond the stimulus and was at times associated with isolated epileptic spikes in the pretectum and pulvinar.

Two stereotaxic HF lesions were made in the left dorsolateral tegmentum. The depth electrodes were not removed after surgery in order to carry out postoperative EEG recordings and stimulation.

POSTOPERATIVE STIMULATION AND EEG RECORDINGS (5 DAYS POSTOPERATIVE)

Five days postoperatively, left midbrain lesion stimulation was done. No responses could be elicited from the electrode in the dorsolateral tegmentum. Stimulation of the mesial tegmentum still produced the fearful sensation in the face. It was concluded that the spontaneous pain had been activated from neural elements in the dorsolateral tegmentum, and, although the mesial region was functionally intact, it was the source for her original pain.

The immediate effect of the lesion was a loss of upward gaze, nystagmus retractorius, an increase in the analgesia over her right face, arm and chest, with lessening of the pain and a disappearance of the hyperesthesia. The facial tic ceased. The patient still felt the "cold" sensation in her arm, but it was not as unpleasant. The intention tremor of the right arm was reduced markedly, with a reduction of the spasticity in her right arm and leg. Hand coordination was slightly better and her gait improved.

Summary of Clinical Observations in the Three Patients

1. Central pain can originate from spontaneous or stereotaxically induced lesions of the dorsolateral portion of the midbrain. Electrical stimulation of these midbrain regions activates the spontaneous pain, and a stereotaxic lesion in the same region will reduce it. Unpleasant sensations can be evoked from the mesial midbrain (periaqueductal region), but the sensations do not have the characteristics of the spontaneous central pain (Fig. 11-9).

2. Spontaneous and/or evoked epileptic activity, such as spikes and spike after-discharges, have been recorded following stimulation of the dorsal midbrain, pretectum and pulvinar in the three patients with central pain. The epileptic phenomena may or may not be associated directly with the patients' spontaneous pain.

3. The facial tic in patient S. M. was activated by electrical stimulation of the dorsolateral tegmentum and it ceased following the therapeutic HF lesion. A facio-ocular seizure associated with epileptic spikes recorded from the pretectum and pulvinar electrodes resulted from midbrain stimulation. Both sensory and motor phenomena which out-

Spontaneous and Induced Phenomena From Midbrain in Central Pain

Patient	Locus of Electrodes	Sensory	Motor	Electrical
No. 1 V. H. Vascular lesion thalamus-midbrain	Dorsolat. tegmentum collicular level	Spontaneous facial pain Induced facial pain with stimulation		Epileptic discharges Epileptic discharges and after-discharges
No. 2 P. B. Trauma Parietal lesion Midbrain lesion	Dorsolat. tegmentum pretectal			Epileptic after-discharge from activation of caudal midbrain
	Dorsolat. tegmentum collicular level	Induced central pain in arm Pain persists (15-30 sec.) beyond stimulus		
No. 3 S. M. Thrombosis thalamus-midbrain	Dorsolat. tegmentum collicular level	Induced facial pain	Activates facial tic	Epileptic after-discharge spread from dorsolat. tegmentum into pulvinar

Figure 11-9. Summary of spontaneous and induced phenomena from midbrain in central pain.

lasted the stimulation were evoked by electrical stimulation of the midbrain.

DISCUSSION

Hughlings Jackson (10) defined epilepsy as a sudden excessive local discharge of gray matter in the CNS. He also described epileptic seizures which he believed originated from various cortical or subcortical regions in his patients. Penfield and Jasper (22) have defined the epileptic discharge as "not only an excessive activation of groups of neurons in the CNS, but an abnormal paroxysmal discharge usually hypersynchronous as well as excessive and usually self-sustained, once precipitated by various activating agents." The EEG recordings from depth electrodes in the midbrain of patients with central pain have revealed epileptic activity occurring in some instances concomitantly with the patients' paroxysms of pain or with sensory and motor phenomena following the period of

electrical stimulation in association with epileptic spikes recorded at rostral sites in the tectum and thalamus. These findings suggest that the
dorsolateral mesencephalon may be the site of development of hyperirritability and epileptic phenomena which, under certain conditions, result in pain. Potentially, all gray regions in the CNS may become hyperirritable, but certain regions of the brain possess an innate hyperirritability and a low convulsive threshold. For example, the hippocampal
cortex has a low threshold of epileptic excitability, while the parietal
cortices possess a higher threshold. Experimental evidence in animals
reveals definite localized differences of regional excitability in the subcortex (2, 13, 23). The neurons of the brain stem reticular formation can
be activated by injections of chemicals, and clonic and tonic convulsions
have been produced chronically in cats following the injection of cobalt
into the mesencephalic tegmental reticulum (20). Sensory phenomenon
owing to localized hyperirritability of the sensory thalamus was noted in
cats after they had been given an injection of strychnine into the sensory
thalamus. The cat was also hypersensitive to peripheral stimuli, and
paresthetic disturbances were reported (7). Less is known about the innate irritability of the brain stem neurons in man. Stimulation in the
subcortex of man has resulted in epileptic after-discharges recorded from
the fields of Forel, the ventrobasal complex of the thalamus and the
dorsolateral midbrain tegmentum (29). Penfield and Jasper (22) point
out the close relationship between convulsive movements and electrical
after-discharge when they arise in the motor cortex. They also report
that even with electrically discharging neurons in the motor cortex, no
movements may occur. One of our patients developed a facio-ocular
seizure with an epileptic after-discharge recorded in the pretectum and
pulvinar electrodes following stimulation of the midbrain. There was
also evidence that in one patient the epileptic spike activity was associated with her facial pains, while in another man no epileptic disturbance
was recorded when the pain was evoked by midbrain stimulation, although his pain persisted beyond the period of stimulation, which suggests the possibility of an after-discharge occurring at some point beyond
the recording electrode in the midbrain.

The origin of the central pain in these three patients was produced by
a spontaneous pathologic lesion at thalamic-midbrain level. Vascular occlusion is a common cause of these lesions. Scarring occurs in any area of
the brain which has been injured, as long as enough circulation is preserved to provide for reaction and reorganization. Injury results in the
destruction of neurons and the outgrowth of neuralgia. Penfield's (22)
studies of the cortical cicatrix revealed an intermediate zone bordering
the scar which was visualized by an anastomatic system or arteries. He

believes that a progressive focal destruction of this intermediate zone results in progressive atrophy of gray matter with a gradual enlargement of the epileptogenic focus. The pathophysiologic response of the brain stem to focal vascular injury is not well known, but a similar pathologic response may occur to produce a scar in the brain stem similar in nature to the cortical scar and capable of becoming epileptogenic. Although the spontaneous lesions in the brain stem that result in central pain are usually due to a vascular insult, trauma such as that produced by a therapeutic midbrain tractotomy may result in a severe dysesthesia (14). The location, type of lesion and local response of brain tissue to trauma may determine whether or not a zone of hyperirritability develops. The pathologic reaction of the brain stem to physical injuries produced by cutting, freezing or heating is not well understood. The open midbrain tractotomy done by cutting the lateral edge of the mesencephalon was often followed by a painful dysesthesia, a factor responsible for the abandonment of the operation (14, 28). On the other hand, thermal lesions seem to result in a lower incidence of this complication (19, 25). Further studies are needed to compare the immediate and long-term effects of various physical injuries to the brain stem and their relationship to the possible development of hyperirritable phenomena.

If central pain, under certain circumstances, is epileptic in origin it would fit Gastaut's (8) concept of a partial epilepsy. He states that a partial epilepsy can occur as a localized epileptic disturbance resulting in a clinical seizure (sensory, motor or experiential). It is due to a focal epileptic hyperirritability and it may remain localized for its duration or, after a time, spread in the brain and become generalized. Gastaut (8) points out the importance of afferent stimulation on local brain tissue hyperexcitability in partial epilepsy. Even the arrival of a normal volley of afferent stimuli may precipitate epileptic activity. The dorsolateral tegmentum is rich in afferent connections with convergence of multiple sensory inputs, which could be one factor responsible for the development of a hyperirritable site in the midbrain. The afferent stimulation in patients with central pain may result in hyperesthesia and hyperalgesia (Case 2 [P. B.] and Case 3 [S. M.]). In these patients the effect was reduced after a therapeutic lesion in the dorsolateral tegmentum. High frequency electrical stimulation of the pain pathways in the spinal cord or brain stem of man has been effective in evoking painful sensations and reproducing certain kinds of central pain (18). Becker *et al.* (1), recording patterns of single cell units in the periaqueductal gray and mesencephalon tegmentum, found evidence of convergence of large and small fiber systems. They concluded that "the summation of peripheral stimuli into a prolonged and increasing central response is one of the characteristics of reaction to stimuli of sufficient intensity to be noxious."

If central pain can, under special circumstances, originate from an irritable epileptic zone bordering on the edge of the pathologic midbrain lesion, is there additional clinical evidence in man for other kinds of hyperirritability phenomena which may be originating from the brain stem (27)? Hughlings Jackson (10), in 1902, described a truncal seizure in a 17-year-old girl that began with fixation of the chest and progressed to involve the arms. He believed this originated in the brain stem or lowest level. Jackson called this seizure a "trunk fit or lowest level fit" and he speculated that it originated at the bulbopontal level. Symonds (26), in 1929, reported a 37-year-old female who developed seizures that began with a feeling of numbness of the fingertips followed by spasms of the tongue. Later, twitching of the left eyelid and side of the mouth occurred, with attack spreading to involve the whole left side of the face and raising of her eyebrows. The attacks were thought by Symonds to be epileptiform, arising from pontobulbar regions, but he ventured no comment as to etiology or pathology. Tonic seizures associated with disseminated sclerosis were recorded by Matthews in 1958 (15). He reported four patients with an unusual sensory and motor seizure pattern. The onset of attacks was rapid, of brief duration and with great frequency in each of the persons. The seizure began unilaterally in the face, arm and leg in three patients and only in the arm of the fourth. There was a rapid spread of the tonic spasm and the seizures appeared to be precipitated by movement, sensory stimulation or hyperventilation. The attacks were extremely painful in three patients, but only a tickling sensation was experienced by the fourth person. There was no direct evidence as to the site responsible for the central lesions or their nature and possible central mechanisms. However, Matthews was of the opinion that the attacks were associated with lesions in the mesencephalon and he regarded the seizures as "focal epileptic fits originating in such lesions." Two of his patients showed immediate improvement when given anticonvulsant medication. He pointed out the importance of the provocation of the attacks by peripheral stimulation, indicating again the importance of an activation of the seizure by afferent stimulation. He also believed that the sensory loss in these patients was attributable to lesions of the spinothalamic tracts. Penfield (21) described in one patient autonomic seizures caused by a tumor compressing the diencephalon. He called them diencephalic seizures, and this observation must have influenced his later thinking in regard to the concept of the centrencephalic seizures.

In 1920, Cushing (5) reported five persons with a syndrome called "painful tic convulsif." The person afflicted was suddenly seized with contractions of the facial muscles and pain (Fig. 11-10). Cushing pointed

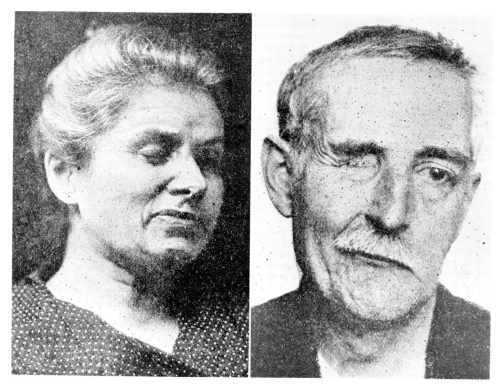

Figure 11-10. Photographs reproduced from Cushing's paper showing facial expression in patients with "painful tic convulsif." Cushing postulated a central origin for the syndrome. Compare with Figure 11-11.

out that the syndrome should not be confused with trigeminal neuralgia, and at the time he postulated a central origin for the paroxysmal facial pain. One of our patients (Case 3 [S. M.]) with central pain also exhibited a facial tic that was activated along with her pain by stimulation of the midbrain. After the therapeutic midbrain lesion, the pain and tic were abolished.

The facial expressions in the patients with spontaneous painful facial tic and the facial expressions in patients and animals resulting from midbrain stimulation bear a strong resemblance (Fig. 11-11). Activation of the central gray area in man and animals results in a complex set of responses including facial and oral movements, autonomic reactions, changes in respiration and unpleasant fearful sensations (6, 18). The central gray area of the midbrain is a region for integration of certain facial sensations and oral reflexes related to sucking and chewing. The autonomic changes are due to activation of the hypothalamic pathways in this midbrain region. Tic douloureux of cranial nerve origin has certain clinical features suggestive of a paroxysmal seizure of a central origin. The pain of the

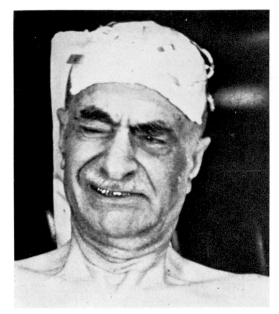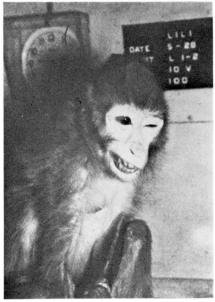

Figure 11-11. Facial expression in patient 2 (P. B.). Central pain from parietal and midbrain lesions. Stimulation of the region adjacent to central gray. Other photograph shows monkey in Delgado's experiment during central gray stimulation. Also see Figure 11-10.

facial tic usually has a sudden focal onset of the paroxysms described by the patient as "stabs of lightning" or "electric shocks." The pain may be triggered by afferent stimulation such as stroking the skin of the face in the region of the referred pain. Persons with multiple sclerosis may develop facial pain thought to be due to the presence of pathologic plaques involving the trigeminal pain pathways in the brain stem. We have relieved a patient with facial pain associated with multiple sclerosis by making a lesion in the mesial portion of the dorsolateral tegmentum, probably interrupting the ascending pain pathways in the quintothalamic tract. King (12) has presented impressive evidence from experiments on animals for a possible central origin of trigeminal tic pain. He and Barnett (11) reproduced a trigeminal tic syndrome in cats by injecting alumina gel into the descending spinal tract of the trigeminal nerve. Crue and Sutin (4) also advocated a central origin for tic pain and other central pain phenomena. Despite the possible central origins of these facial pains, anticonvulsant drugs have not been effective in giving relief.

The oculogyric crises of parkinsonism may result from a hyperirritable phenomenon originating in the tectum of the mesencephalon. The tectal region is an essential synaptic region for the integration of conjugate ocular movements (18, 19). The neural regions responsible for conjugate eye movements are adjacent to the pain pathways in the dorsal midbrain and may also be susceptible to similar pathophysiological changes responsible for hyperirritability. Stimulation of the pretectum in one patient with central pain (Case 3 [S. M.]) resulted in a complex facio-ocular seizure, with upward eye deviation and the occurrence of epileptic spikes in the pretectum and pulvinar. Recently Shanzer and coworkers (24) reported a twenty-year-old woman with seizures induced by deviation of her eyes. Depth electrode recording in this patient from the temporal, occipital and frontal lobes revealed no epileptic focus. She died, and at postmortem examination no cause for the seizures could be found. Shanzer and his associates postulated: "The possibility cannot be ruled out that these seizures originated in the depth of the brain—namely the paramedian region of the left midbrain and pretectum."

Clinical and electrographic evidence of a hyperirritability in the region of the dorsolateral midbrain tegmentum was found in three patients with central pain. These observations are still incomplete due to a lack of anatomical confirmation regarding the exact extent and nature of the pathophysiologic process in the midbrain and the exact localization of the recording electrodes. Further clinical observations in man are surely needed. It is now feasible and safe to evaluate patients with central pain by using advanced neurophysiological techniques employing electrodes implanted chronically in the midbrain. The neurophysiologist must join the clinician in crossing the animal experimentation gap and evaluating human suffering with pain. Direct observations made in man continue to be of prime importance if we are to increase our understanding of pain. This view was emphasized by Hardy, who stated "the verbal report of the instructed subject is the most reliable evidence that the pain threshold has been reached" (9).

REFERENCES

1. BECKER, D. P.; GLUCK, H.; NULSEN, F. E., and JANE, J. A.: An inquiry into the neurophysiological bases for pain. *J Neurosurg,* 30:1, 1969.
2. BERGMANN, F.; COSTIN, A., and GUTMAN, J.: A low threshold convulsive area in the rabbit's mesencephalon. *Electroenceph Clin Neurophysiol* 15:638, 1963.
3. CASSINARI, V., and PAGNI, C. A.: Central Pain: *A Neurosurgical Survey.* Cambridge Mass., Harvard, 1969.
4. CRUE, B. L., JR., and SUTIN, J.: Delayed action potentials in the trigeminal system of cats. *J Neurosurg* 16:477, 1959.
5. CUSHING, H.: The major trigeminal neuralgias and their surgical treatment based on experiences with 332 gasserian operations. The varieties of facial neuralgia. *Amer J Med Sci,* 160:157, 1920.
6. DELGADO, JOSE M. R.: Cerebral structures involved in transmission and elaboration of noxious stimulation. *J Neurophysiol* 18:261, 1955.
7. DUSSER DE BARENNE, J. G.: Central levels of sensory integration. *Sensation: Its Mechanisms and Disturbances.* Baltimore, Williams & Wilkins, 1935.

8. GASTAUT, HENRI and FISCHER-WILLIAMS, M.: The physiopathology of epileptic seizures. *Handbook of Physiology.* Washington, D.C., American Physiological Society, 1959, Vol. I.

9. HARDY, T. D.; WOLFF, H. G., and GOODELL, H.: *Pain Sensations and Reactions.* Baltimore, Williams & Wilkins, 1952.

10. JACKSON, H.: Observation of a case of convulsions (trunk fit or lowest level fit). In Taylor, James (Ed.) *Selected Writings of John Hughlings Jackson.* New York, Basic Books, 1958, Vol. I.

11. KING, R. B., and BARNETT, J. C.: Studies of trigeminal nerve potentials. Overeaction to tactile facial stimulation in acute laboratory preparations. *J Neurosurg,* 14:617, 1957.

12. KING, R. B.: Evidence for a central etiology in tic douloureux. *J Neurosurg,* 26:175, 1967.

13. KREINDLER, A.; ZUCKERMAN, E.; STERIADE, M., and CHIMION, D.: Electroclinical features of convulsions induced by stimulation of brain stem. *J Neurophysiol,* 21:430, 1958.

14. McKENZIE, K. G.: *Trigeminal Tractotomy Clinical Neurosurgery.* Baltimore, Williams & Wilkins, 1955.

15. MATTHEWS, W. B.: Tonic seizures in disseminated sclerosis. *Brain,* 81:193, 1958.

16. MULLAN, S.; HARPER, P. V.; HEKMATPANAH, J.; TORRES, H., and DOBBEN, G.: Percutaneous interruption of spinal pain tracts by means of strontium 90 needle. *J Neurosurg,* 20:931, 1963.

17. NASHOLD, B. S., JR., and WILSON, W. P.: Central pain. Observations in man with chronic implanted electrode in the midbrain tegmentum. *Confin Neurol,* 27:30, 1966.

18. NASHOLD, B. S., JR.; WILSON, W. P., and SLAUGHTER, D. G.: Sensations evoked by stimulation in the midbrain of man. *J Neurosurg,* 30:14, 1969.

19. NASHOLD, B. S., JR.; WILSON, W. P., and SLAUGHTER, D. G.: Stereotaxic midbrain lesions for central dysesthesia and phantom pain. *J Neurosurg,* 30:116, 1969.

20. NEEDHAM, C. W., and DELA, C. J.: Cobalt epilepsy and the reticular formation. Abstract presented American Academy of Neurology Meeting, April 1969.

21. PENFIELD, WILDER: Diencephalic autonomic epilepsy. *Arch Neurol (Chicago),* 22:358, 1929.

22. PENFIELD, W., and JASPER, H.: *Epilepsy and the Functional Anatomy of the Human Brain.* Boston, Little, 1954.

23. RALSTON, B. L., and LANGER, J.: Experimental epilepsy and brain stem origin. *Electroenceph Clin Neurophysiol,* 18:325, 1965.

24. SHANZER, S.; APRIL, R., and ATKIN, A.: Seizures induced by eye deviation. *Arch Neurol (Chicago),* 13:621, 1965.

25. SPIEGEL, E. A., and WYCIS, H. T.: Mesencephalotomy for relief of pain. In: Anniversary Volume for O. Poetzl, Vienna: 1948.

26. SYMONDS, C. P.: Epileptiform attacks, apparently of ponto-bulbar origin. *Proc Roy Soc Med,* 22:597, 1929.

27. STERLING, W.: Le type spasmodique telanoide et tetaniforme de l'encephalite epidemique remarques sur l'epilepsie "extra-pyramidale." *Rev Neurol (Paris),* 31 (ii): 484, 1924.

28. WALKER, A. E.: Relief of pain by mesencephalic tractotomy. *Arch Neurol (Chicago),* 48:865, 1942.

29. WILSON, W. P., and NASHOLD, B. S., JR.: Epileptic discharges occurring in the mesencephalon and thalamus. *Epilepsia (Amsterdam),* 9:265, 1968.

Chapter 12

TRIGEMINAL PAIN

RICHARD BLACK*

THE numerous attempts to define the mechanism involved in paroxysmal trigeminal neuralgia, or tic douloureux, and the multiplicity
of treatments available for patients with this condition indicate that there
is little understanding of this syndrome. Of the current theories concerning this state, and other pain states of apparent central origin, the one
most closely fitting the data presented in this paper is that these alterna-
tions of sensory modality are in some way related to a central pool of
neuronal hyperactivity, or epileptic focus (6, 12). The apparent relationship between epilepsy and certain paroxysmal pain syndromes such as trigeminal neuralgia, tabes dorsalis and even paroxysmal abdominal pain is
not a new concept. It has been recognized since the time of Trousseau
(17), who described tic douloureux as epileptiform neuralgia. Subsequently, Kinnier Wilson (20) described the trigeminal neuralgia paroxysm
as the result of sensory epileptiform discharges. More currently, Crue
(6-9) has presented further evidence of this.

The clinical similarities of paroxysmal dysfunction of the sensory system to epilepsy, as seen, for example, in patients with trigeminal neuralgia, herpes zoster and other pain states of central origin, are indeed most
striking. These similarities include the nature of sudden onset of pain,
abrupt cessation of the paroxysm and functional consistency of the region
involved. Recent recordings of epileptic units in the thalamus of patients
with facial pain and recordings of epileptic units in the spinal cord of
patients with segmental pain following traumatic partial amputation of
the cord add more credence to the view that an epileptic focus in the
sensory system may be related to paroxysmal pain-like states. Unfortunately, not as much is known about the central pathophysiology of these

* It is impossible to list here all of the individuals who, through their writings, personal
communications or collaboration have contributed over the past eight years to the ideas presented in this paper about epilepsy and deafferentation and their possible relation to the
understanding of some pain states in human beings. The personal encouragement and contributions of the late Dr. Jerzy Olszewski, Dr. Jacob Abraham of Velore, India, and Dr. A. A. Ward,
Jr. of Seattle must, however, be noted. This work is presently being continued by Dr. L. E.
Westrum of the Departments of Biological Structure and Neurological Surgery and Dr. R. C.
Canfield of the University of Washington School of Dentistry in collaboration with the present
author.

This work was financed in part by Public Health Service Grant #NB-04053 and GSRF 171,
FAC RES.

119

pain states because the patients yield no clear EEG abnormalities on
scalp recordings and the clinician must principally rely on symptoms, not
signs, for his analysis of the disease.

Epilepsy, in the presently accepted clinical definition of the word, implies a paroxysmal discharge in the central nervous system that is expressed by an alteration of motor function or of the level of consciousness
or both. Here, clinical observation, the use of the EEG and microelectrode
recording have demonstrated, in many cases, a relation between clinically
observable manifestations of this disease and a localized hyperactivity in
the central nervous system. If a similar relationship exists between paroxysmal pain states and such localized central hyperactivity, it should
also be demonstrable.

This attempt to relate paroxysmal pain states and focal central nervous
system hyperactivity is divided, for clarity, into three parts. The first of
these is concerned with the effect of various experimental epileptic foci
placed systemically at several different locations in the nervous system of
cats and monkeys. Very different behavioral effects, some indeed pain-like,
are related to the different anatomical locations of essentially similar epileptic foci or localized groups of hyperactive neurons. In the second part,
supporting evidence from studies of human beings is reviewed very briefly.
Neuronal hyperactivity is often found associated with pain states of central
origin. The third part is intended to answer the question, If localized
neuronal hyperactivity is associated with paroxysmal pain states of central
origin, what then is the possible etiology, in the human being, of these
areas of central neuronal hyperactivity and what etiology is common to all
the many proposed causes of trigeminal neuralgia?

Part I: Effects of Location of the Epileptic Focus

The experimental work reported here was designed to explore the hypothesis that paroxysmal pain-like states are related to a central localized
region of neuronal hyperactivity similar to that found in individuals who
have focal motor epilepsy. This was done by systematically placing experimental epileptic foci at various different locations in the nervous system and, after observing the behavioral response of the animal, verifying
by recordings and histologic studies that an epileptic focus has indeed
been created at a given site.

To date, a total of 189 cats and three monkeys have been used. A
single epileptic focus was produced in each animal, under a relatively
short-acting anesthetic, at a single discrete location in the nervous system.
Thus, each animal demonstrated the effect of a solitary epileptic focus of
known location and character. The criteria for these epileptic foci were
that they be localized functionally for a reasonable period of time so that

TABLE 12-I

EPILEPTOGENIC AGENTS

Epileptogenic agents used to produce localized neuronal hyperactivity in various locations in the central nervous system. The majority of the lesions were made using the first two agents listed.

Tungstic Acid Gel	Penicillin
Alumina Gel	Strychnine
Alumina Oxide	Tetanus Toxin
Cobalt	

(Tungstic acid gel was employed because of the convenient time of its course (4). Alumina gel was used to produce more chronic lesions that lasted a year or more.)

observed behavioral effects might be ascribed to them and that neuronal hyperactivity might be demonstrated in the appropriate area by micro-electrode recordings. Functional localization means that the behavioral effects observed could be related, according to our current understanding of the function of the nervous system, to the anatomical site of the epileptic focus as localized by histologic studies and microelectrode recordings. Epileptic neuronal hyperactivity was considered to be present at a location when the autonomous firing rates observed were greatly in excess of those found normally at this location in control animals, and this activity was expressed in paroxysms similar to those seen in the cerebral cortical focus where it has been described in association with focal motor epilepsy (18).

These epileptic foci were produced by injection of a very small amount of one of several epileptogenic agents (Table 12-I). Depending on the physical characteristics of the agent used, the injections were made by means of microsyringes through broken-off glass micropipettes or #27 needles. The agents used were tungstic acid gel, alumina gel, aluminum oxide, cobalt, penicillin cream and dilute tetanus toxin. All of these agents consistently produced focal motor epilepsy when injected into the sensori-motor cortex of cat or monkey, thus demonstrating their epileptogenic properties in the classic sense. The epilepsy produced by all of these agents was characterized by a latent period followed by a building up of the epileptic type of activity to a maximal level. Except for different time courses and maximal intensity of action, the results obtained were independent of the agent used. The time course of the various agents appeared to be independent of the site of injection if a constant quantity of the agent was injected. Latent periods extended from a few hours with tungstic acid gel to a month or more with alumina gel. The most intense effects both behaviorally and when using neuronal hyperactivity as a measure were produced by tetanus toxin. The least intense and most chronic effects were caused by alumina gel. The effects of these 0.01 to 0.02 ml injections cannot be compared directly with the effects of the

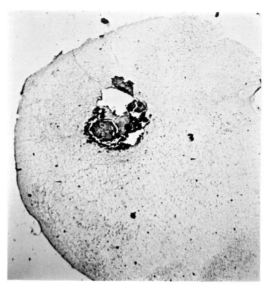

Figure 12-1. Cross section of cat brain stem at level of closed medulla. A large tungstic acid focus is shown in the spinal nucleus of the trigeminal nerve at the level of the caudal part of pars interpolaris.

much larger quantities used by other investigators to produce cortical motor epilepsy. Over 40 percent of the animals in this series were treated with tungstic acid gel because of its convenient pattern of rapid action. The lesions were clearly defined histologically (Fig. 12-1) and the physiological effects were recorded (Fig. 12-2).

The behavioral effects produced by localized epileptic foci placed in various parts of the nervous system were also investigated systematically (Fig. 12-3). Animals with injections of epileptogenic material into peripheral nerve, dorsal root ganglion, dorsal columns, the descending spinal trigeminal tract, and the trigeminal dorsal root and the gasserian ganglion exhibited no behavioral changes long after the epileptogenic agent would have been expected to have acted. Furthermore, no neuronal hyperactivity around the site of the injection was found in microelectrode examinations of these animals. Since histologic studies verified the site of injection in the above-mentioned structures, it was concluded that the epileptogenic agents used did not produce neuronal hyperactivity in tissue that lacked central gray matter.

All the animals in our series that were given injections of epileptogenic material into various parts of the central grey matter demonstrated some behavioral response. Furthermore, all of these animals (over 130) demonstrated localized neuronal hyperactivity similar to that seen in cerebral cortical epilepsy.

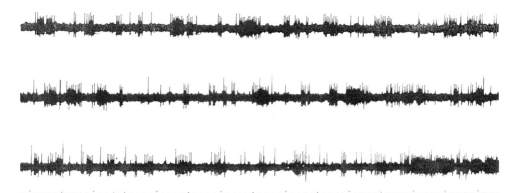

Figure 12-2. Neuronal hyperactivity produced by injection of alumina gel into pars caudalis of the spinal trigeminal nucleus. The injection of 0.02 ml of the autoclaved alumina gel reconstituted with saline was made 162 days previously. The animal had exhibited tic-like signs involving the second and third divisions of the trigeminal nerve on the side ipsilateral to the injection for approximately 100 days prior to the recording above. Recording made with 1 megohm saline-filled micropipettes under conditions of drug-induced paralysis and regional anesthesia. This area, in the absence of an epileptic focus or deafferentation would exhibit no spontaneous activity under these conditions. Time marks are 10, 50 and 100 milliseconds.

Animals receiving injections of epileptogenic material into the tip of the dorsal horn of the spinal cord would start to excessively groom the dermatomal segment involved at about the time neuronal hyperactivity began. In cats, which groom by licking, the whole dermatome would soon be denuded of hair and the skin reddened. At this time, an over-action characteristic of avoidance or withdrawal was readily elicited by touching the segment or by lightly blowing on it. As the central epileptic focus developed, following the time course characteristic of the epileptogenic agent used, the animal would begin to demonstrate more severe involvement of the sensory system. Paroxysmal attacks, lasting ten to fifteen seconds, would occur two to twenty minutes apart. These were apparently spontaneous in nature, with no discernible eliciting stimulus; but, when a puff of air or a light touch was applied to the dermatomal segment involved an attack was evoked readily, providing that the stimulus was not applied immediately following an attack. Light touch was much more effective in provoking a seizure than was heavy pressure. At this stage of development of the epileptic focus, the animal would sit between paroxysms—neither sleeping nor eating. During paroxyms, the animal would exhibit violent activity, destructively biting or scratching the part of its body involved. It should be emphasized that this activity was not a patterned motor response.

A species difference between cat and monkey became apparent. The

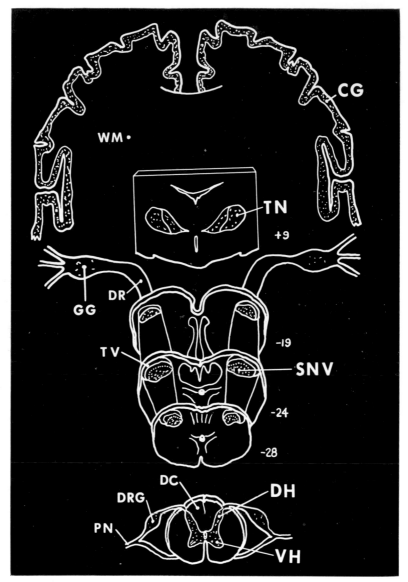

Figure 12-3. Schematic diagram of nervous system showing selected sites of injection of an epileptogenic agent. The sites shown by the smaller letters on the left of the diagram were made into peripheral nerve, dorsal root, gasserian ganglion or central white matter. In all of these situations neither neuronal hyperactivity nor behavioral changes were observed. The sites indicated by the larger letters on the right were made into some form of central gray matter and all resulted in localized neuronal hyperactivity and behavioral changes appropriate to the site of the injection. CG—cortical gray; DC—dorsal columns; DH—dorsal horn; DR—dorsal root; DRG—dorsal root ganglion; GG—gasserian ganglion; PN—peripheral nerve; SNV—spinal nucleus of the fifth nerve; TN—thalamic nuclei; TV—descending spinal tract of the fifth nerve; VH—ventral horn; WM—white matter. Numerals indicate coordinates in mm.

cat viciously bit and clawed the affected part of its body during the paroxysms; while the monkey, in contrast, tended to explore the area involved or later actually avoided touching it, while vocalizing or clutching around the periphery of the area. Both cat and monkey gave clear evidence that they had a sensory problem that involved all of their attention. (As an extension of the description in the text, a movie accompanied the presentation of this material at the City of Hope Symposium on Pain and Suffering. This movie emphasized the different behavioral responses produced in both cats and monkeys by various differently located epileptic foci. The movie began with an example of simple focal motor epilepsy with no apparent sensory involvement and concluded with segments of film following the time course of the development of trigeminal neuralgia-like signs in a monkey.)

Animals with a similar epileptic foci located in the ventral horn of the spinal cord had localized paroxysmal motor activity appropriate to the segment involved, without any great sensory involvement and certainly without apparent concern between paroxysms. No excessive grooming or other attention was paid to the dermatome involved. For example, a cat with a developed epileptic focus in ventral horn of the lumbar spinal cord might have a tonic-clonic seizure of its right hind limb while drinking milk from a dish. The cat would turn around, look at the limb, remain balanced on the remaining three limbs and continue drinking, demonstrating a patterned localized motor response with minimal sensory involvement.

Injections of epileptogenic agents into the spinal nucleus of the fifth nerve always produced marked overreaction to facial stimulation on the ipsilateral side. A marked exaggeration of the five to five and the five to seven reflexes became apparent early in the development of the focus. This gradually developed into spontaneous paroxysmal facial spasms. At this time the animal's reaction to a touch on its face became more dramatic and, if the central focus was small, a localized peripheral area very sensitive to touch could be demarked. The animal characteristically gave a very positive avoidance reaction to anything approaching or touching its face. These paroxysmal facial spasms, similar to spinal cord paroxysms, were triggered readily by light touch or draft. During the paroxysms induced by a fully developed lesion, the pupils dilated, respiration became rapid and there was often vocalization. Each of the paroxysms, occurring ten to fifteen minutes apart, might last for ten to fifteen seconds and result in violent but nonpatterned motor activity. Cats characteristically groomed the affected side of the face during development of the central focus. As the seizure activity peaked, cats clawed destructively at the face. Monkeys, which explored the face with their fingers during development of the cen-

tral focus, later avoided touching the area involved, often clutching around
the periphery or rubbing the homologous area on the opposite side. Neither
species slept nor ate between paroxysms. The animals appeared to have all
attention occupied completely by their sensory problem. No patterned
motor behavior accompanied the paroxysms.

Sites where epileptogenic material was to be injected into the thalamus
were selected by electrical stimulation of the face, and placement of the
injecting needle depended upon a maximal response recorded previously
in sensory thalamus. Several interesting, bizarre behavior patterns resulted
from foci in this area. Occasional clonic movements were observed in limbs
opposite to the side of the lesion. These were apparently without any
"pain-like" sensations. Often the animals exhibiting these clonic movements stared into space and drooled after cessation of the movement.
Sometimes generalized convulsions and loss of consciousness resulted, after
which the animal exhibited a complex pattern of motor behavior. One
animal with a lesion in the sensory thalamus demonstrated obstinate progression, walking into and pushing against obstacles like a wall, radiator or
table. According to the observers, these animals groomed the side opposite
to their epileptic focus more than they normally did. Electroencephalo-
graphs of two of these animals showed characteristic three-second spike and
wave activity reminiscent of the petit mal epilepsy pattern in human beings.
It should be emphasized that no apparent strong sensory involvement
resulted from thalamic lesions, and the seizure pattern in each animal was
individualistic. No further attempt was made in this study to document
behavior patterns in relation to the site of lesion, because our primary
interest was in pain states of central origin.

Injection of the sensory cortical gray matter in the somatosensory area
resulted in little alteration in behavior between paroxysms of seizure
activity. This type of activity was characterized by focal motor seizures
involving part of the opposite side of the body. Occasionally the seizure
spread, becoming generalized. No hyperaesthesia or evidence of altered
sensory function could be detected in these animals. The observations of
Penfield (16) that pain in human beings usually does not accompany
cortical epilepsy are of interest in light of our observations.

The majority of the above-cited examples resulted from rather intense
epileptic foci produced by the shorter-acting agents. A milder effect resulted
from small epileptic foci made with alumina gel, a longer-acting agent, in
the spinal trigeminal system. Of the animals treated with this substance
three have been kept alive for longer than a year. Each has developed a
similar behavior pattern that has resulted in avoidance of contact with
the affected side of its face. No changes were noted until three months
or more after the injection had been made. Then over a period of two

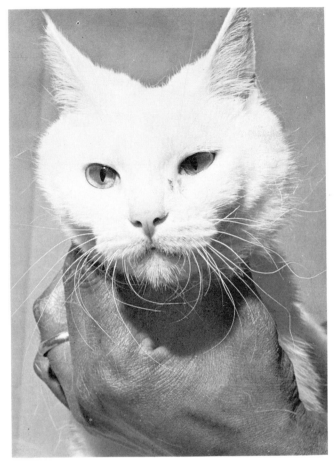

Figure 12-4. Cat received an injection of alumina gel into the left spinal nucleus of the fifth cranial nerve 9 months before photograph was taken. Behavioral responses related to the first and second divisions of the trigeminal nerve had been noted for 5 months. Note the lack of care on the left side of the face and the irregular pattern of the left vibrissae.

to three months, each animal began to avoid contact with the side of its face ipsilateral to the injection. When this side of the face was deliberately touched or rubbed, the animal would then retire to a corner of the room and excessively groom that side of its face for the ensuing three to five minutes. The affected side of the face usually showed lack of care. The hair and eye were not cleansed and there was kinking and curling of the whiskers (Fig. 12-4). Spontaneous paroxysms were observed on the affected side of the face, apparently related to some sensory abnormality. These might occur only once every two to three hours. At that time any ongoing activity would cease and the animal would concentrate its

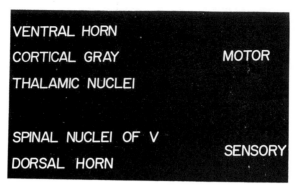

Figure 12-5. Schematic division of sites of epileptic foci in the nervous system showing those producing paroxysmal patterned motor activity and those producing paroxysmal sensory aberration.

full attention on the affected side of the face. These paroxysms can be so demanding as to stop an animal in a midair leap.

Study of results of injection of epileptogenic agents into 189 cats and three monkeys revealed that no animal with ventral horn, cortical or thalamic foci had a primary sensory problem and, conversely, no animal with a focus in the trigeminal nucleus or the dorsal horn exhibited a patterned motor response (Fig. 12-5). *There appears to be a level of demarcation in the ascending sensory system above which epilepsy presents itself as a primary motor phenomena and below which it is an intense paroxysmal aberration of the sensory system.*

Part II: Suggestion of Neuronal Hyperactivity Accompanying Pain States in Human Beings

It has been demonstrated experimentally that an epileptic focus can, when properly located, produce a paroxysmal pain-like state in animals, but epileptic-like neuronal activity at appropriate sites in human beings suffering paroxysmal clinical pain has not yet been directly demonstrated. At present, there is only indirect evidence relating neuronal hyperactivity to paroxysmal pain states of central origin.

A central pool of neuronal hyperactivity is suggested by the recording of efferent (antidromic) activity from the human peripheral trigeminal nerve during a paroxysm of trigeminal neuralgia by Crue (8). Similar spontaneous antidromic activity had been shown by King (12) to be related in animals to paroxysms of an epileptic focus located in the central trigeminal complex. The epileptic type of activity reported by Nashold (14), originating in the midbrain of patients having facial pain, has been described in Chapter 11. His findings are further evidence that there is a pain-related epileptic process located at the more primary sensory levels. The demonstration by microelectrode recording of epileptic-like neuronal hyperactivity following chronic deafferentation of the human spinal cord and its possible relation to diffuse episodic pain has been reported by Loeser (13).

In addition to evidence obtained by direct electrical recordings from the nervous system, the implication of the success obtained in treating patients with pain of central origin with anticonvulsant drugs such as Dilantin (11) and Tegretol (5) cannot be ignored when considering the question of whether an epileptic-like state accompanies central pain in the human.

Part III: Etiology of Neuronal Hyperactivity in the Sensory System

So far we have shown that experimental epileptic foci in the primary nuclei of the ascending sensory system of animals can produce such an intense sensory aberration that it seems justified to call this a pain-like state. We have also considered some tentative evidence that epileptic activity has been found to accompany some pain states in man. The possible etiology of epileptic activity, even focal epileptic activity, in the sensory system at levels that produce pain-like states must now be considered.

The effect of massive deafferentiation of a sensory system, such as retrogasserian rhizotomy in the trigeminal system, is of interest. Clinical results of this procedure have been evaluated in the ten-year follow-up postrhizotomy series reported by Pete and Schneider (15). Three-hundred eighty-two patients were included in the study (Table 12-II). None of the resulting paresthesias resembled the lancinating trigeminal neuralgias for which the rhizotomies were originally done. Instead, these paresthesias were more diffuse and not as paroxysmal in nature. This unexplained after-effect of rhizotomy led to a laboratory investigation in which the cat was used as the experimental animal.

The purpose of the experiments, reported in detail elsewhere (1), was to learn whether a central mechanism caused paresthesias to occur after rhizotomy. It was also hoped that additional information would be obtained about the behavior of neurons within the central nervous system

TABLE 12-II

TEN YEAR FOLLOW-UP POSTRHIZOTOMY SERIES OF PEET AND SCHNEIDER (15)

Number of patients	382	
Paresthesias		
Crawling-Drawing	213	(55.7%)
Burning	116	(30.4%)
Numbness	16	(4.1%)

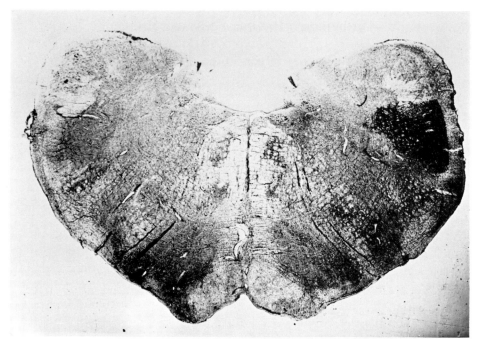

Figure 12-6. Nauta stain of cross section of cat brain stem at level of obex eight days after trigeminal rhizotomy. Note the intense localized area of degeneration.

following deafferentation (2). An extradural transtemporal trigeminal rhizotomy was done with the aid of the Zeiss operating microscope on one side of each surgically anesthetized animal. These animals had been previously examined for evidence of facial or head trauma, and the condition and age of the teeth were noted. At selected times, from one to thirty-five days following rhizotomy, microelectrode recording was done in the locally anesthetized animal paralyzed with gallamine or curare. Rectal temperature, femoral arterial blood pressure, pulse rate, respiratory rate and PCO_2 of the expired air were monitored throughout each experiment to insure that a near-normal physiological state of the animal was being maintained. Recordings from the nondeafferentated side of the brain stem were similar to those previously recorded in this laboratory under similar conditions from animals with intact trigeminal nerves. These data were therefore considered as individual control data for each animal in the series. Recordings of neuronal activity in the experimental cats from pars interpolaris and pars caudalis of the deafferentated spinal trigeminal nucleus, on the side ipsilateral to the rhizotomy, demonstrated with time the development of grossly abnormal spontaneous hyperactivity resembling that seen in epilepsy. This occurred in areas showing histological changes characteristic of deafferentation.

Histological sections of the brain stem revealed that complete trigeminal rhizotomy consistently resulted in a high degree of degeneration that was confined to the localized anatomical area of the descending spinal tract and nucleus of the fifth nerve (Fig. 12-6). More detailed examination of the area by use of the electron microscope demonstrated dense degenerated presynaptic bags that were seen at all survival times, but were most numerous at three to six days after rhizotomy (Fig. 12-7). It was noted that the middle member of serial synapses was affected by the rhizotomy when these were involved in the degeneration. Electron microscopic examinations showed that the primary afferent endings mainly contact dendrites directly, and in turn receive an axo-axonic synapse from another source; possibly cerebral cortex or interneurons (19). This arrangement possibly forms the structural basis for the presynaptic inhibition demonstated in this anatomical area (10).

Extracellular recording, using glass micropipettes filled with 3M KCl or NaCl, from the above-described areas of deafferentation showed the progressive development of epileptiform activity. At the same time, recordings from the intact or control side uniformly showed a lack of any

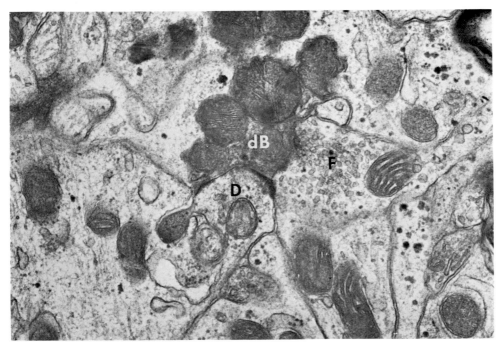

Figure 12-7. An electron micrograph taken from the spinal trigeminal nucleus (pars interpolaris) three days after ipsilateral retrogasserian rhizotomy. A dense, degenerated ending (dB) synapses with a dendritic profile (D) and receives a synaptic contact from a normal ending containing "flat" synaptic vesicles (F). Magnification ×25,000.

spontaneous neuronal activity in the spinal trigeminal complex. Evoked responses of single cells to peripheral stimulation were readily obtained and appropriate to the peripheral stimulus.

The time course of the development of this epileptiform activity is of interest. For the first one to two days following rhizotomy, recordings from the deafferentated spinal complex appeared similar to those from the intact side except, of course, no response to peripheral nerve stimulation was obtained. Between two and ten days after rhizotomy, spontaneous low-frequency discharges resembling that phenomenon described by physiologists as "synaptic noise" appeared through the entire deafferentated nucleus. During the six weeks these animals were followed, this progressed into an almost continuous high-frequency discharge (Fig. 12-8). The pattern of firing is quite similar to that recorded from epileptic foci in both man and monkey. Occasionally, burst-like firing patterns were observed to emerge from the continuous ongoing activity (Fig. 12-9). Following this, autonomic changes such as pupil dilation and an increase in blood pressure were observed in the animal. Waves that were synchronous with unit bursting were recorded from the cortex and thalamus. The continuous high-frequency discharge, which in some cases occurred continuously between paroxysms of burst-like firing patterns, was

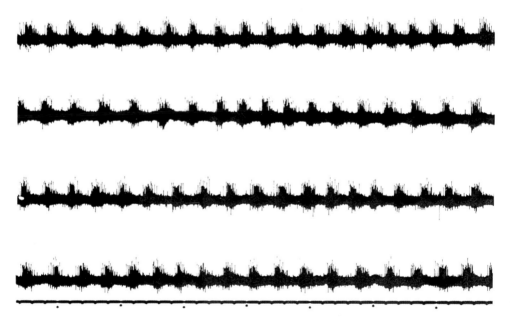

Figure 12-8. Neuronal hyperactivity recorded from the pars interpolaris of the spinal trigeminal nucleus of cat deafferentated 19 days previously by transtemporal retrogasserian rhizotomy. Recording from 3 molar KCl-filled glass micropipettes in a regionally anesthetized paralyzed cat preparation. Time marks are 100, 500 and 1000 milliseconds.

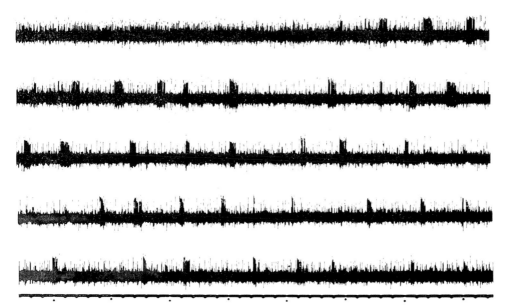

Figure 12-9. Neuronal hyperactivity recorded from the pars interpolaris of the spinal trigeminal nucleus of cat deafferentated 31 days previously by transtemporal retrogasserian rhizotomy. Note the transition from continuous ongoing activity, left top tracing, to an intermittent bursting type of pattern. This transition was followed by autonomic changes in the animal and evidence of propagation of the bursting wave form to higher centers. Recording from 3 molar KCl-filled glass micropipettes in a regionally anesthetized paralyzed cat preparation. Time marks are 100, 500 and 1000 msec.

not related to any activity in cortex or thalamus that could be detected using the same techniques. Evidence of axonal propagation beyond the deafferentated nuclei but within the brain stem of this neuronal hyperactivity was an occasional finding.

It has been shown that neuronal hyperactivity develops in the deafferentated trigeminal complex in the cat following total retrogasserian rhizotomy. Various aspects of this hyperactivity are of possible clinical interest. There is a latent period following rhizotomy before the development of hyperactivity. The development of the hyperactivity is preceded by an increase in lower frequency background activity. This is soon followed by extremely rapid bursts of unit discharges. The nature of the gradual onset suggests an adaptive physiological and possibly anatomical change occurring in the deafferentated neurons. This correlates well with the clinical state, since there is always a delay seen following surgery before the patient develops paresthesia. Some clue as to whether the hyperactivity recorded in the deafferentated part of the brain stem is consciously perceived is suggested by the propagation of the pattern of bursting of this discharge activity and the reception of this pattern at the cortical level. The significance of this is not yet known.

While total deafferentation has been shown to produce a massive central degeneration and a diffuse sensory paresthesia, the effects of partial deafferentation are clinically much more interesting. Removal of the teeth produces a localized partial deafferentation of the trigeminal system as well as a localized hyperactivity, which in turn interacts with the adjacent intact sensory pathways. Exploration of the spinal trigeminal complex with microelectrodes thirty days after total extraction of the teeth from one side of the head reveals small areas of neuronal hyperactivity medial and ventral in the spinal complex. These areas are relatively as epileptic as the whole tract was following deafferentation, but are anatomically much more localized (3). The localization corresponds to areas from which direct tooth pulp afferents may be recorded in the intact animal. In addition to localized hyperactivity, an alteration of the central response to stimulation of the skin of that side of the face occurs. Prolonged after-discharges occurring at intensity levels very close to the stimulation threshold and lasting up to thirty or more seconds are found on the side from which teeth had been extracted (Fig. 12-10). Refinement of this technique to the extent that only the pulp of the teeth is extracted has given similar physiological results and, in addition, shown resulting central degeneration in the appropriate areas (Fig. 12-11). The

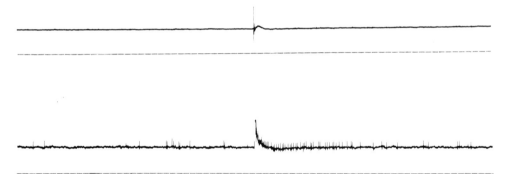

Figure 12-10. *Top Tracing:* Response of cells in spinal nucleus of the fifth nerve to electrical stimulation of the skin of the ipsilateral upper lip applied through bipolar needles spaced 3 mm apart. The stimulus was well above threshold. *Bottom Tracing:* Response of cells from the homologous area on the opposite side of the same animal. The stimulus was applied ipsilateral to the side of recording in an identical manner but at threshold level. Thirty days before recording, the teeth of the upper and lower jaws had been extracted from this side. Note the ongoing spontaneous activity to the left of the stimulus and the prolonged after discharge following even a threshold stimulus. Stimulus, 0.01 millisecond pulse recording from 3 M KCl-filled glass micropipettes; preparation paralyzed and regionally anesthetized, normal body temperature and expired CO_2. Time marks 10, 50 and 100 milliseconds.

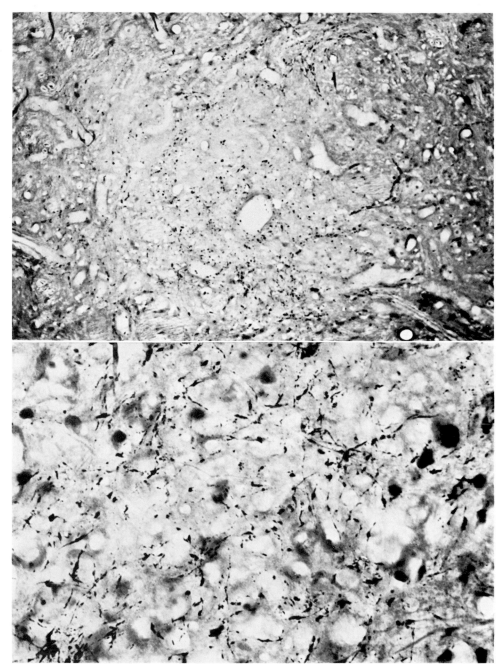

Figure 12-11. *Top:* Low magnification light micrograph of a Nauta-gyax stained preparation, showing degeneration in the spinal trigeminal nucleus (pars interpolaris) 10 days after ipsilateral tooth pulp removal. The degeneration is not distributed evenly but it is concentrated in the ventral regions of the nucleus and is also seen contralaterally. Magnification approximately ×500. *Bottom:* A higher magnification micrograph of a preparation similar to that shown in Figure 12-11A, detailing the character and density of degeneration products. Magnification approximately 2500×.

135

effect of partial deafferentation in the trigeminal system is now being studied by a team composed of Dr. Robert C. Canfield, School of Dentistry of Washington; Dr. Lesnick E. Westrum, Department of Neurological Surgery, University of Washington; and the author. Efforts are being made to correlate electron microscopic observations and physiological studies of the central effects of tooth pulp extraction and loss of other specific neuronal receptors in the spinal trigeminal system. More complete understanding of the trigeminal sensory system may well contribute to the development of better means for treating patients with intense sensory aberrations.

In conclusion; first, it has been demonstrated that experimentally induced epileptic foci in the gray matter of the primary afferent system produce intense paroxysmal sensory aberrations that occupy all of an animal's attention. The aberration can reasonably be termed a pain or pain-like state. Second, in some pain states in humans, epileptic-like units have been reported previously by others. Third, central neuronal hyperactivity may be produced by peripheral deafferentation. This hyperactivity acts to distort sensory input from adjacent intact pathways in experimental animals.

The possible clinical significance of these findings must be considered in relation to pain states of central origin. Many different etiologies have been proposed for the cause of trigeminal neuralgia. The one factor that appears in all of the reasonable hypotheses is that some neuronal damage has occurred peripherally or centrally. The thesis postulated here is that this neuronal damage, no matter how produced, will result in changes in related areas of gray matter in the central nervous system. In some susceptible individuals these changes can result in a paroxysmal pain state of central origin. That the nature of these gray matter changes is epileptic is suggested by the experimental work presented in this paper.

REFERENCES

1. ANDERSON, L.; BLACK, R. G.; ABRAHAM, J., and WARD, A. A., JR.: Deafferentation neuronal hyperactivity—a possible etiology of paresthesias following retrogasserian rhizotomy. Presented at 1967 meeting of American Assoc. of Neurological Surgeons. (Manuscript presently submitted for publication.)
2. BLACK, R. G.; ABRAHAM, J., and WARD, A. A., JR.: Afferent system epilepsy and paroxysmal pain-like states. (Manuscript in preparation.)
3. BLACK, R. G.; WESTRUM, L. E., and CANFIELD, R. C.: Focal central deafferentation and neuronal hyperactivity produced by dental lesions. (Manuscript in preparation.)
4. BLACK, R. G.; ABRAHAM, J., and WARD, A. A., JR.: The preparation of tungstic acid gel and its use in the production of experimental epilepsy. *Epilepsia (Amsterdam)*, 8:58, 1967.

5. BLOM, S.: Tic douloureux treated with new anticonvulsant. *Arch Neurol (Chicago),* 9:285, 1963.
6. CRUE, B. L.; SHELDEN, C. H.; PUDENZ, R. H., and FRESHWATER, D. B.: Observations on the pain and trigger mechanisms in trigeminal neuralgia. *Neurology (Minneap),* 6:196, 1956.
7. CRUE, B. L., and SUTIN, J.: Delayed action potentials in the trigeminal system of cats. Discussion of their possible relationship to tic douloureux. *J Neurosurg,* 16:477, 1959.
8. CRUE, B. L.; CARREGAL, E. A., and TODD, E. M.: Neuralgia; considerations of central mechanisms. *Bull Los Angeles Neurol Soc,* 29 (3):107, 1964.
9. CRUE, B. L.; TODD, E. M., and CARREGAL, E. A.: Cranial neuralgia—neurophysiological considerations. In Vinken, P. J., and Bruyn, G. W. (Eds.): *Handbook of Clinical Neurology,* vol. 5. Amsterdam, North Holland Publishing Co., 1968.
10. DARIAN-SMITH, I., and YOKOTA, T.: Cortically evoked depolarization of trigeminal cutaneous afferent fibers in the cat. *J Neurophysiol,* 29 (2):170, 1966.
11. IANNONE, A.; BAKER, A. B., and MORRELL, F.: Dilantin in the treatment of trigeminal neuralgia. *Neurology (Minneap),* 8:126, 1958.
12. KING, R. B.; MEAGHER, J. N., and BARNETT, J. C.: Studies of trigeminal nerve potentials in normal compared to abnormal experimental preparations. *J Neurosurg,* 13:176, 1956.
13. LOESER, J. D.; WARD, A. A., JR., and WHITE, L. E., JR.: Chronic deafferentation of human spinal cord neurons. *J Neurosurg,* 29 (1):48, 1968.
14. NASHOLD, B. S., JR.; WILSON, W. P., and SLAUGHTER, D. G.: Sensations evoked by stimulation in the midbrain of man. *J Neurosurg,* 30:14, 1969.
15. PEET, M. M., and SCHNEIDER, R. C.: Trigeminal neuralgia. A review of six hundred and eighty-nine cases with a follow-up study on sixty-five per cent of the group. *J Neurosurg,* 9:367, 1952.
16. PENFIELD, W., and JASPER, H.: *Epsilepsy and the Functional Anatomy of the Human Brain.* Boston, Little, 1954.
17. TROUSSEAU, A.: *Clinque Medicale de L'Hotel-Dieu de Paris; ed. 5.* Paris, J. B. Bailliere et fils, 1877.
18. WARD, A. A., JR.: The hyperexcitable neuron-epilepsy. In Rodahl, K., and Issekutz, B., Jr. (Eds.): *Nerve as a Tissue.* New York, Harper, 1966.
19. WESTRUM, L. E., and BLACK, R. G.: Changes in the synapses of the spinal trigeminal nucleus after ipsilateral rhizotomy. *Brain Res,* 11:706, 1968.
20. WILSON, K.: *Neurology.* Baltimore, Williams & Wilkins, 1940.

Chapter 13

A NEUROPHYSIOLOGICAL EXAMINATION OF CENTRAL PAIN MECHANISMS

Donald P. Becker

RECENT years have seen advances in both the clinical management of patients with pain problems and the development of sophisticated methods of examining the fine anatomy and electrical activity of the nervous system. Information concerning central nervous pathways and connections, as well as electrophysiological responses, has improved our understanding of basic mechanisms in sensibility. However, there still remains a great gap in our ability to define the structures and mechanisms that are characteristic of the central determinants of pain.

Is Pain a Modality?

The question of modality specificity in pain mechanisms represents a major area of controversy. In its purest form, the specificity theory suggests that stimulation of specific individual cutaneous receptors (which provide sensation for only one modality) results in central conduction of nerve impulses in specific peripheral fibers that project to specific central and anatomically distinct pathways in spinal cord and brain (19, 32).

This concept of a direct telephone line nervous system involving focal modality representation continues to be applied to the interpretation of pain phenomena. An intense search for pain receptors and nociceptive fibers has been made in the past and continues. Although there is little doubt that free nerve endings and small fibers in nerve and anterolateral spinal cord are important in the recognition of noxious stimuli, small fiber receptors with very high thresholds are found infrequently. Unmyelinated C fibers $(0.5\text{-}1.5\mu$ in diameter), originally considered along with the smaller myelinated delta axons to be pain fibers, have been shown to have a variety of receptors specifically and exquisitely sensitive to cold or to warmth or to touch (11, 12). It thus appears that the large number of unmyelinated fibers (which in cutaneous nerves outnumber myelinated fibers 3 to 12 times) (31) subserve various modalities just as do the myelinated fibers. Iggo (13) has stated that the great majority of afferent unit small myelinated fibers are excited by quite mild mechanical stimulation, so that nociceptors in this range of fiber sizes must form only a small proportion of the total sample. Although he found more high threshold receptors when examining the unmyelinated C fibers, again the large majority were excited by innocuous stimuli. More recently, Perl (22) noted that 20 percent of myelinated fibers examined in primate skin required mechanical stimuli for activation. These were the smaller fibers, and he considered those responding only to noxious deformation as nociceptors.

Since pain is such a ubiquitous phenomenon, this relative lack of very high threshold units suggests that, although some receptors may have significantly higher thresholds than others, the concept of specific nociceptor receptors and fibers can be misleading. Pain is not a modality like touch, temperature, vision or audition. Rather, pain should be defined as an intensity phenomenon. Excesses of any of the specific modalities, i.e. temperature extremes or excessive pressure, may result in pain perception. As Noordenbos (21) has suggested, pain is "too much."

The search for specific nociceptors, nevertheless, has certainly been fruitful. It has demonstrated some degree of specificity in many receptors, but not infrequently receptors demonstrate more than one type of adequate physiological stimulus. For example, they may respond both to pressure and temperature changes. Such findings support the concept that spatial and temporal discharge patterns must be important to the organism for modality discrimination.

Further evidence that pain should be considered an intensity phenomenon and not a modality comes from peripheral nerve stimulation experiments. With increasing strength of electrical stimuli to the exposed and electrically monitored sural nerve in the human being during experimentation, any parameters of stimulation resulting in pure large fiber activity never gave rise to sensations described as painful. Pain was expressed at the moment delta fiber activity was noted with increased stimulus. Pain was also experienced with isolated small fiber activation after large fiber activity was blocked (7, 8). Such data have been used to suggest that there is an important relationship between fiber size and the transmission of sensation that is judged to be painful.

Small fibers certainly are crucial to pain transmission, but great care must be taken in interperting these results. Firstly, the biophysical nature of peripheral nerve fibers is such that lower intensity electrical stimulation excites the large fibers, and the smaller the fibers the stronger the stimulus needed for excitation. This does not mean that the receptors themselves follow the same response gradation to physiological stimuli. Thus, very low levels of electrical stimuli (less than 0.5 volts) were used for pure large fiber (B fiber) stimulation. Much stronger intensities were required to excite the smaller myelinated delta fibers and poorly myelinated C fibers. Secondly, it has not been proven that maximal and intense pure large fiber peripheral stimulation will not cause pain because it has not as yet been possible to do this without also stimulating delta fibers.

Furthermore, although low-level stimulation of the posterior columns in man may have an inhibitory effect on pain perception, Sweet *et al.* (29) have reported that stronger levels of stimulation to this rapidly conducting, larger-fibered system in man will cause a markedly unpleasant sensation. The author has recently stimulated the dorsal columns of a patient under local anesthesia. At low levels of stimulation the patient described lessening of the pain of a pinprick or pinch to his lower extremities. At higher levels of stimulation, however, the stimulus itself was considered quite noxious and the patient asked that it not be repeated. The "electric shock" sensation was referred caudally and, therefore, it was not considered to be due to local root stimulation.

Thus, the concept of specific nociceptors, specific pain fibers and specific pain tracts can be misleading. Pain may better be considered an intensity phenomenon related to complex central inhibitory and excitatory events resulting from the type and strength of the stimulus.

Mesencephalic Response Patterns Related to Graded Peripheral Stimuli

The author and his colleagues (3) have recently studied response patterns of single units extracellularly in medial mesencephalon. In this study they were concerned not only with the presence or absence of a response in a given unit, but in its response pattern which might correlate with information about intensity, as increasing peripheral electrical or physiological stimuli were applied through gradations considered non-noxious to reach noxious levels. The medial mesencephalon of cats was chosen as the locus of recording for the following reasons: First, the anterolateral quadrant of the spinal cord projects to this area (4, 14, 20) and has been recognized as important in the transmission of painful stimuli since the time of Gowers (1878) (10), a fact confirmed frequently when anterolateral cordotomy is performed to relieve pain. Second, stimulation of the smaller fibers in the peripheral nerve results in activity in this region (6), and the smaller fibers are of critical importance in the perception of pain (7). Third, the larger fibers of the dorsal column have been found to terminate lateral to this region (24), and interaction between these two systems may be important in those central events following peripheral stimuli that lead to pain perception. The region studied extended within these Horsley-Clarke coordinates: anterior 2.0 to 4.0; lateral 1.0 to 2.0; depth 2.0 to −4.0. This included periaqueductal gray and ventral tegmentum.

Supramaximal trains of electric stimuli were applied at three to five second intervals to the pads of the forepaws alternately as the electrode was being advanced down a track. Any unit responding to this stimulus was then examined, providing the spike duration was greater than 200 μsec. Stimulation was then applied to the superficial radial nerve and recordings were obtained in the following manner: one hundred consecutive 0.5 msec stimuli just above A-beta (A large), just above A-beta-gamma-delta (A large and small), and just above A + C thresholds were applied at 4.25 second intervals. The one hundred responses of the peripheral nerve and central unit at each level of stimulation were recorded on magnetic tape. Physiological stimulation was usually applied in separate experiments, but occasionally in the same experiment with the distal exposed nerve left intact. Touch and rub were considered non-noxious. Pinch was applied with a hemostat and heat was applied with a focused flood lamp. Physiological stimuli were first applied for two seconds after a five second delay to determine response frequency, and then through one minute periods for interspike interval analysis.

It is of interest that of over one hundred units observed, only 25 percent did not respond grossly to electrical forepaw pad stimulation. One hundred and twenty units were held long enough to perform a complete analysis. A unit responding to forepaw stimulation on one side almost always responded similarly to stimulation on the opposite side, but the response was generally more intense on one side than the other. The few exceptions to bilateral response came in neurons that responded only to large fiber stimulation, and the responding neuron was usually on the opposite side from the stimulus.

The units responding to peripheral nerve electrical stimulation had characteristic response patterns that could be classified into specific groups:

Type I. (Response to A-beta alone, short latency [5 to 10 msec] and short duration [20 to 50 msec] response [18% of total]. Figure 13-1 is an example of a unit in this group, in this instance devoid of spontaneous activity. As one hundred responses were averaged, the Y axis represents the number of discharges per stimulus. The three graphs represent the response pattern just above the three different thresholds for A large (A-beta), A (A-beta-gamma-delta) and A + C. With increasing stimulus intensity the response pattern was essentially the same, but the total number of discharges per stimulus increased slightly. The latency to the first response was 8.75 msec, suggesting that several synapses were crossed before this central neuron was excited. This unit responded only once or twice to each 0.5 msec shock, but most units in this group fired two to four times to each stimulus.

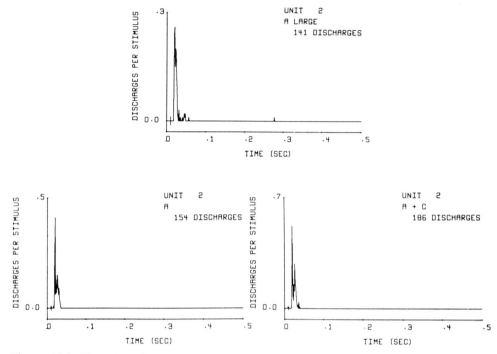

Figure 13-1. Type I unit (A 4.0, L 1.0, D –0.9). The ordinate represents number of discharges per stimulus as 100 responses were averaged. The stimulus artifact is represented by the small vertical line at a 10 msec delay. The response pattern is essentially the same with increasing stimulus intensity, but the total number of discharges increases.

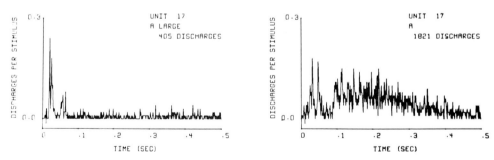

Figure 13-2. Type II unit (A 3.0, L 1.0, D –1.1). At A-beta there is an early burst beginning at 6.25 msec and a second smaller burst from 42.5 to 55.0 msec after the stimulus. With stimulation at the delta level the smaller second burst becomes larger, and after an 83.75-msec delay there begins a prolonged burst of increased firing lasting as long as 390 msec. The increased base line activity relates in part to the "wind-up" effect described in the text.

Type II. (Response to A-beta as in Type I, plus a second response of long duration [350 msec or more] appearing with A-beta-gamma-delta activation [32%].) Figure 13-2 shows a unit in this group responding to A-beta with a latency of 6.25 msec. There is a second smaller burst of activity from 42.5 to 55.0 msec after the stimulus at this level. It is not possible to determine whether this represents the multiple firing pattern of this unit to A-beta stimulation or whether slower conducting fibers (such as A-gamma) were also stimulated peripherally and caused this later response. When the peripheral nerve stimulus was raised to bring in A-delta, a prolonged burst of activity resulted, beginning 83.75 msec after the stimulus and lasting out to 390 msec. This prolonged burst of increased firing was not correlated with blood pressure changes.

Type III. (No response to A-beta only, but response to A-beta gamma-delta, long latency [up to 500 msec], very long duration [3 to 4 sec and longer] [27%].) Units in this group did not respond to A-beta stimulation, as shown in Figure 13-3. At the delta level in this unit, after a 500 msec delay there is a rather marked progressive increase in firing up to a maximum at 1.2 seconds. This continues for six seconds, after which it slowly declines back to the baseline after twelve seconds. In this instance, because of the long duration response at the delta level, only ten consecutive stimuli were given and analyzed at thirty-five second intervals. Two other units in this group responded over a very long duration lasting more than eight seconds, and the remainder had increased firing lasting up to three to four seconds. The long delay again suggests that multiple synapses are crossed before the midbrain neuron is stimulated.

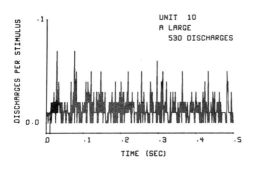

100 Added Responses

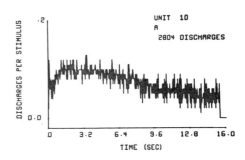

10 Added Responses

Figure 13-3. Type III unit (A 4.0, L 1.5, D –2.5). There is no significant response at A-beta level. At A-beta-gamma-delta there is a marked increase in firing, reaching a maximum at 1.2 msec, continuing at this level for 6 sec and declining to the base line after 12 sec. This prolonged response was not correlated with blood pressure.

Type IV. (Response as in Type II or III, but when C added, a very late burst of activity from 1.3 to 2.5 seconds after the stimulus [13%].) Within the limits of the technique utilized, the addition of C activation by the peripheral nerve stimulus did not strikingly change the response pattern over that seen with total A fiber activation. Often, however, the total number of discharges increased. In addition, there occasionally occurred a very late burst of activity between 1.3 and 2.6 seconds after the stimulus.

Type V. (Inhibition of spontaneous activity at A-beta or A-beta-gamma-delta threshold, usually with short latency [10%].) Spontaneous activity of units in this group was inhibited either at A-beta-gamma-delta levels of stimulation. These units rapidly and progressively became silent with repeated stimulation and were not subjected to computer analysis.

The pattern of response of neurons to A large and A large plus small fibers was noted to be different in another way. Type I neurons responding only to A-beta did not change their frequency or duration of re-

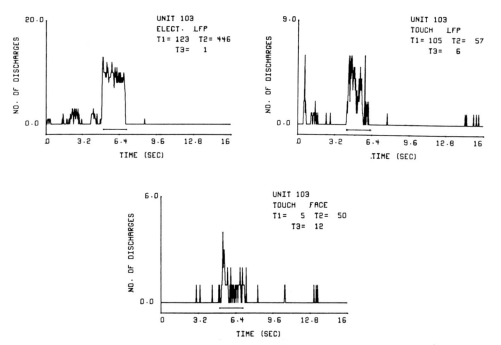

Figure 13-4. (A 3.5, L 1.0, D –1.7). In this single 16 sec record, stimulation was applied for 2 sec after a 5 sec delay. There is a short latency response with no other discharge to supramaximal electric shock and touch. When these units responded to noxious stimuli, the response pattern was similar. T_1 represents number of discharges in the prestimulus period, T_2 the stimulus period and T_3 the post-stimulus period.

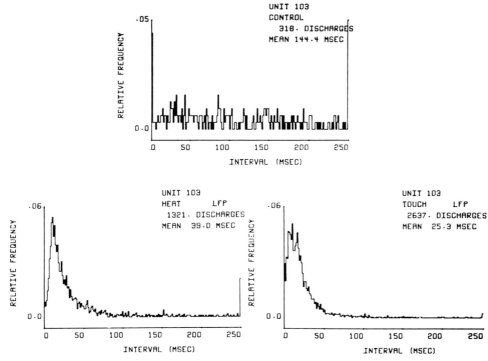

Figure 13-5. Interspike interval record from unit shown in Figure 13-4. There is a response to touch and to heat, but the mean interval is shorter and the number of discharges greater with touch.

sponse with each subsequent stimulus. However, Type II, III, and IV neurons responding to A-beta-gamma-delta with a prolonged response often displayed a progressive increase in frequency and duration of response with each subsequent stimulus, until the cell would fire continuously at a rate much higher than had occurred spontaneously. This "wind-up" has been described by Mendell (18) in the dorsolateral column of the cat spinal cord with stimulation of C fibers in a peripheral nerve.

Response patterns to physiologic stimuli often demonstrated similarities to those seen with electrical peripheral nerve stimuli. Those units which responded to non-noxious stimuli (30%) generally had short duration responses with little or no after-discharge. When the stimulus became intense, little change was noted in the response. Figure 13-4 illustrates an example. This is a single sixteen second record, and the stimulus, represented by the horizontal line, was applied after a five second delay. There is a short latency increase in firing to a supramaximal two second electric shock to the left forepaw pad. There is no after-discharge and, in point of fact, there is poststimulus inhibition. Units responding in this fashion (with short latency and no after-discharge) characteristically responded identically to a non-noxious stimulus such as touch. If they responded to mechanical noxious stimuli, the pattern was similar. That these units often had wide peripheral fields is demonstrated by the response seen to touch to the left face.

Figure 13-5 is an interspike interval record of the same unit taken from a sixty second record of spontaneous activity, of response to heat and of response to touch. This unit responded both to touch and to heat, but with a shorter mean interval and greater response to touch than to heat.

In contrast, those units responding primarily to noxious stimuli (60%) demonstrated a prolonged after-discharge. Figure 13-6 gives an example. The long after-discharge to a supramaximal electrical stimulus and small response to touch is noted. Figure 13-7 is an interspike interval record of this unit. There is a definite increase in firing and shortening of the interspike interval with intense heat, whereas with prolonged touch there is some inhibition as the number of discharges diminish and the mean interval increases. This inhibition of firing with prolonged touch was found in more than 90 percent of the primarily noxious responding neurons analyzed.

The mode of central response to physiological stimuli could be predicted from the response observed to a two second supramaximal electrical stimulus. Units that responded with a short latency and short duration were primarily touch responders; units responding with short latency and prolonged duration responded both to touch and noxious stimuli, but to noxious stimuli with a prolonged discharge; units responding with long latency and long duration responded mainly to noxious stimuli with a prolonged discharge. Thus, physiologic stimuli appeared to exhibit variations in unit response analogous to those observed in the Type I, II and III responses to electrical peripheral nerve stimulation.

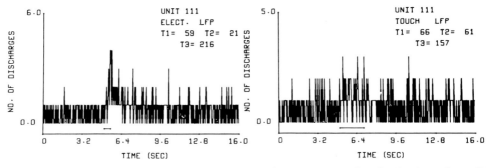

Figure 13-6. (A 4.0, L 1.0, D +0.7). A prolonged response to electric shock and small response to touch is illustrated in this unit.

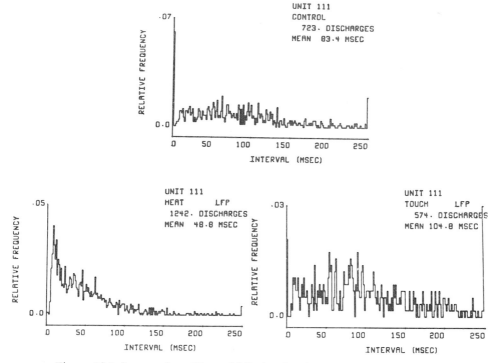

Figure 13-7. Same unit as Figure 13-6, showing interspike interval record.

It was also observed that neurons responding to noxious stimuli with a long duration response would also frequently show the "wind-up" effect with repeated noxious stimuli. Those responding primarily to non-noxious stimuli without an after-discharge only rarely showed the "wind-up" with any type of stimulus.

No separate topographical or anatomical organization of differently responding units could be determined in this study. Units demonstrating each major pattern type were found admixed in periaqueductal gray as well as in ventral tegmentum.

Peripheral Intensity and Central Summation Concept of Pain

Recent studies have demonstrated that there is convergence of both myelinated and unmyelinated peripheral axons upon a single secondary sensory neuron in the spinal cord (18) (23). It has been shown that a single axon in the dorsolateral column of the cat may respond to both. A fiber stimulation and C fiber stimulation, and to each in a very different way. Thus, the cable theory becomes suspect as soon as peripheral neural impulses are transmitted across the first central synapse. Furthermore, as noted above, certain single midbrain neurons are responsive to both large and small fiber stimulation. This has also been observed by Amassian and DeVito (2).

Other important interrelationships between the large fiber system and smaller fiber system have been demonstrated. It has been suggested that the large fiber system has an inhibiting effect on the smaller fiber system, and a theory of pain mechanisms has been presented based on these concepts (15, 16). This theory holds that large fiber sensory input has an inhibiting effect, beginning at the first central synapse, upon the small fiber system. This concept has been used to explain pain problems such as postherpetic neuralgia and tabes dorsalis, where large fibers have been damaged out of proportion to small fibers (21).

There can be no doubt that small fibers in nerve and in the antero-lateral spinal cord are important in the recognition of noxious stimuli. But the problem remains that small fibers in the anterolateral system subserve non-noxious sensations as well, so that their activity may not signal pain. Rather, we must look for a pattern or code within this system that relates to pain perception.

The author and his associates have shown that moderately distinctive types of response to intense electrical stimulation can be demonstrated in single neurons in the medial mesencephalon and that natural or physio-logical stimuli that are judged to be painful or noxious give similar responses. Mendell (18) has described similar prolonged responses to A + C fiber stimulation in the dorsolateral column of the cat. She did not, however, subdivide the A fiber input, and in the study described in this paper stimulation of A delta fibers appeared responsible for this mode of central response. Although the duration of the delayed response at C fiber threshold in the cord in the report of Mendell was shorter than those observed in the midbrain in this study, it is noteworthy that it is seen centrally in the spinal cord. Indeed, a prolonged after-discharge in medial spinal cord (25), as well as in medial caudal medulla (5) and midbrain of cat (6), to intense stimuli has been described in experiments employing macroelectrodes.

Our principal interest was in determining the response patterns to the differential peripheral stimuli described, and thus to identify a central correlate possibly related to stimulus intensity. In view of the similarity of the prolonged responses found to nerve stimuli above delta threshold and to noxious physiological stimuli, it is tempting to consider this as a neural response to pain. This possibility becomes more intriguing when we consider the evidence that pain experience occurs in man when the peripheral nerve fiber diameters being stimulated include the smaller gamma-delta group. One might theorize that the prolonged and intense response of multiple units in this region and perhaps in others might signal to the animal that the stimulus is noxious, that pain perception may be related to intensity of neuronal responses and that pain is signaled when this quantitative response reaches a certain level. The "wind-up" effect or increasing central response observed after repeated intense stimuli may relate to this quantitative mechanism.

The concept that pain has no specific receptors, but is produced in the nervous system as a result of summation of impulses excited by intense stimuli is not new. It was suggested by Goldscheider (9) in 1898, and by Sherrington (27) in 1900. Sinclair (28) has indicated that since the paper of Achelis (1) in 1936, little has been heard of the summation theory of pain. This may relate in large part to the fact that the theory was based on clinical intuition without direct neurophysiological evidence. Our findings of long-duration responses and summation of central responses to intense and repeated stimuli provide new support for this theory of central pain mechanisms.

In discussing central mechanisms of cranial neuralgia, Crue and his associates suggested that it might be considered as a consciously interpreted subjective painful phenomenon, probably due to discharge of central internuncial pools in response to many and varied summated stimuli. In 1968, Melzak and Casey (17) proposed the following model for central integration of pain processes: (a) sensory input through the neospinothalamic projection provides, in part, the neurological basis of the sensory discriminative dimension of pain, (b) activation of reticular and limbic structures underlies the motivational drive and unpleasant affect, (c) that higher central nervous system processes exert control over activity in both discriminative and motivational systems. They suggested that the drive mechanisms associated with pain are activated when the input into the reticular limbic system exceeds a critical level. The author would agree with this, having obtained data that tend to support these concepts.

It must be mentioned that demonstrating differential responses in neural units to differential peripheral stimulation is not equivalent to the demonstration that this change has a particular significance to the organism. One cannot necessarily equate central activity upon peripheral small fiber stimulation with pain, because small fibers carry other information. Central activity in this particular locus, moreover, may be related to an alerting phenomenon or an autonomic response.

Stimulation of the Human Anterolateral Spinal Cord

In the course of over fifty stereotaxic cordotomies for intractable pain, the author and his associates have stimulated through the electrode tip after insertion into the cord to aid in target localization. Unlike the findings of Sweet *et al.* (29), there was a very low threshold in the anterolateral system. With the electrode in anterolateral quadrant, low intensity stimulation (0.2 V to 0.5 V, 60 cycles per second) yields most often a tingling sensation in contralateral body. Occasionally a patient mentions a warm feeling in a contralateral site, but rarely a cool sensation. Only when these symptoms are noted will generation of a lesion at safe power levels and for a safe period of time yield contralateral analgesia. Analgesia will begin most densely in the body area defined by stimulation. If the initial area of analgesia is in the leg, this will extend up the body as the lesion is increased, but upward extension may require deeper penetration of the electrode. Conversely, if the initial area affected is the hand, analgesia can be extended down the trunk to include the leg, but this may require withdrawal of the electrode to a more lateral position in the cord.

These findings supply further evidence for a degree of topical arrangement in the anterolateral ascending system (probably primarily in neospinothalamic tract). However, overlap of fiber organization is probably considerable. This is suggested by the fact that differential cordotomy, whereby only the leg, trunk or arm is made analgesic, often results in early regression of the analgesia. In contrast, solid high levels of contralateral analgesia, where the majority of the anterolateral column is destroyed, more often produces long-lasting analgesia. It, therefore, seems desirable to destroy most of the anterolateral quadrant when performing cordotomy, even for pain below the umbilicus.

Of further interest are the symptoms noted by the patient with more intense stimulation (over 0.5 V, 60 CPS) of the anterolateral quadrant. This causes the patient to complain of a disagreeable pain or often a burning sensation covering more of the contralateral body. The patient will usually ask you to stop the stimulus when the approximately 1.0 volt level is reached. In more cooperative patients, if the stimulus is increased further or the frequency increased to over one hundred cycles per second, the burning pain becomes bilateral and may be most intense in the midline abdominal region. This bilateral pain, referred primarily to the abdomen, may be secondary to stimulation of the short-chained more medial propriospinal system. And, once again, the seemingly obvious point is emphasized that increasing stimuli or frequency of stimulation, exciting more fibers and central neurons, results in increasing complaints of pain or severe burning.

Clinical Correlations

The suggestion of Melzak and Wall (16) that large fiber input to the spinal cord may have an inhibitory effect on excitation of central neurons involved in pain transmission has had recent clinical testing. With low level, high frequency dorsal column stimulation, Shealy and Mortimer (26) have demonstrated a 60 to 100 percent elevation of the pain threshold. Sweet and Wepsic (30) have also demonstrated decreased complaints of pain in patients as a result of large fiber peripheral nerve stimulation and dorsal column stimulation.

That inhibitory mechanisms may be taking place, not only at cord level but also at the mesencephalic level, is suggested by the following: It is not infrequently noted that patients with pelvic carcinoma, complaining of unilateral leg pain, will develop significant pain in the opposite leg shortly after cordotomy. With stereotaxic cordotomy performed on the awake, alert patient, this new pain has occasionally been noted to appear immediately, as soon as the lesion is made which results in contralateral analgesia. This suggests not only that inhibitory processes are occurring above the foramen magnum (since the lesion is made at C1-2), but also that inhibitory pathways exist in the anterolateral quadrant as well as in dorsal columns.

Another interesting phenomenon seen in patients with analgesia from cordotomy is referred pain with intense stimulation in the analgesic zone. Patients may often describe the pain as poorly localized, or it may be referred to a contralateral site or be noted just above the analgesic level. White and Sweet (33) have reported that intense electrical stimuli (over 100 V) in the analgesic zone always caused intolerable but poorly described pain in over forty patients that they studied.

Such poorly localized or referred pain supports the concept of the multisynaptic afferent system suggested by Noodenbos (21). Thus, with destruction of neospinothalamic fibers, the usual sensory-discriminative dimension of pain has been blocked, but activation of reticular structures through the paramedial older ascending system, with activity crossing below the level of cordotomy, may still summate to result in pain sensibility, albeit localized inaccurately.

CONCLUSIONS

The following conclusions may be drawn from this report:

1. Considering pain to be a specific modality is misleading. Rather, pain conceptualization may be better defined as an intensity and summation phenomenon related to complex central inhibitory and excitatory events resulting from the type and strength of the stimulus.

2. Small-fibered systems are critical in the transmission of impulses that result in pain perception. Low-level, large fiber stimulation may inhibit this transmission. There is no proof, however, that intense pure

large fiber stimulation will not cause pain under certain circumstances.

3. There is evidence of convergence of both large and small fiber afferent systems on units in medial mesencephalon. In the study reported here, units responding primarily to stimulation that activated small fibers or was noxious, characteristically showed a very prolonged response. In addition, these units often demonstrated a summation effect with repeated intense stimuli. This summation of peripheral stimuli into a prolonged and increasing central response may be one of the characteristics of reaction to stimuli of sufficient intensity to be noxious.

REFERENCES

1. Achelis, J. D.: Die Physiologie der Schmerzen. *Nervenarzt*, 9:559, 1936.
2. Amassian, V. E., and Devito, R. V.: Unit activity in reticular formation and nearby structures. *J Neurophysiol*, 17:575, 1954.
3. Becker, D. P.; Gluck, H.; Nulsen, F. E., and Jane, J. A.: An inquiry into the neurophysiological basis for pain. *J Neurosurg*, 30:1, 1969.
4. Bowsher, D.: Termination of the central pain pathway in man: the conscious appreciation of pain. *Brain*, 80:606, 1957.
5. Collins, W. F., and Randt, C. T.: Evoked central nervous system activity relating to peripheral unmyelinated or "C" fibers in cat. *J Neurophysiol*, 21:345, 1958.
6. Collins, W. F., and Randt, C. T.: Midbrain evoked responses relating to peripheral unmyelinated or "C" fibers in the cat. *J Neurophysiol*, 23:47, 1960.
7. Collins, W. F., Jr.; Nulsen, F. E., and Randt, C. T.: Relation of peripheral nerve fiber size and sensation in man. *Arch Neurol (Chicago)*, 3:381, 1960.
8. Collins, W. F.; Nulsen, F. E., and Shealey, C. N.: Electrophysiological studies of peripheral and central pathways conducting pain. In Knighton, R. S. and Dumke. P. R. (Eds.): *Pain*. Boston, Little, 1966, pp. 34-46.
9. Goldscheider, A.: Uber der Schmerz: Gesammelte Abhandlungen. In *Physiologie der Hautsinnesnerven, Vol. I.* Leipzig, J. A. Barth, 1898.
10. Gowers, W. R.: A case of unilateral gunshot injury to the spinal cord. *Trans Clin Soc, Lond*, 11:24, 1878.
11. Iggo, A.: Cutaneous heat and cold receptors with slowly conducting (C) afferent fibres. *Quart J Exp Physiol*, 44:362, 1959.
12. Iggo, A.: Cutaneous mechanoreceptors with afferent C fibres. *J Physiol (London)*. 152:337, 1960.
13. Iggo, A.: Concluding discussion. In de Reuck, A. V. S., and Knight, J. (Eds.): *Touch, Heat and Pain. Ciba Foundation Symposium*. London, J. and A. Churchill, 1966.
14. Mehler, W. R.; Feferman, M. E., and Nauta, W. J. H.: Ascending axon degeneration following anterolateral cordotomy. An experimental study in the monkey. *Brain*, 83:718, 1960.
15. Melzak, R., and Wall, P. D.: On the nature of cutaneous sensory mechanisms. *Brain*, 85:331, 1962.
16. Melzak, R., and Wall, P. D.: Pain mechanisms: a new theory. *Science*, 150:971, 1965.

17. MELZAK, R., and CASEY, K. L.: Sensory, motivational, and central control determinants of pain: A new conceptual model. In Kenshalo, D. (Ed.): *The Skin Senses.* Springfield, Thomas, 1968.

18. MENDELL, L. M.: Physiological properties of unmyelinated fiber projection to the spinal cord. *Exp Neurol,* 16:316, 1966.

19. MULLER, J.: *Zur vergleichended Physiologie des Gesichtssinnes des Menschen und-der Thiere nebst einem Versuch uber die Bewegungen der Augen und uber den menschlichen Blick.* Leipzig, C. Cnobloh, 1826.

20. NAUTA, W. J. H., and Kuypers, H. G. J. M.: Some ascending pathways in the brain stem reticular formation. In Jasper, H. H.; Proctor, L. D.; Knighton, R. S.; Noshay, W. C., and Costello, R. T. (Eds.): *Reticular Formation of the Brain.* Boston, Little, 1958, p. 3.

21. NOORDENBOS, W.: *Pain.* Amsterdam, Elsevier, 1959.

22. PERL, E. R.: Myelinated afferent fibres innervating the primate skin and their response to noxious stimuli. *J Physiol (London),* 197:593, 1968.

23. POMERANZ, B.; WALL, P. D., and WEBER, W. V.: Cord cells responding to fine myelinated afferents from viscera, muscle and skin. *J Physiol (London),* 199:511, 1968.

24. SCHROEDER, D.; YASHON, D.; BECKER, D. P., and JANE, J. A.: The evolution of the medial lemniscus in primates. *Anat Rec,* 160:424, 1968.

25. SHEALY, C. N.; TYNER, C. F., and TASLITZ, N.: Physiological evidence of bilateral spinal projections of pain fibers in cats and monkeys. *J Neurosurg,* 24:708, 1966.

26. SHEALY, C. N., and MORTIMER, J. T.: Dorsal column electroanalgesia. Presented at meeting of American Assoc. of Neurological Surgeons, Cleveland, Ohio, April, 1969.

27. SHERRINGTON, C. S.: Cutaneous sensations. In Schafer, E. A. (Ed.): *Textbook of Physiology.* Edinburgh and London, Y. J. Pentland, 1900, vol. 2, pp. 920-1001.

28. SINCLAIR, D. C.: *Cutaneous Sensation.* London, Oxford University Press, 1967.

29. SWEET, W. H.; WHITE, J. C.; SELVERSTONE, B., and NILGES, R.: Sensory responses from anterior roots and from surface and interior of the spinal cord. *Trans Amer Neurol Ass,* 165:1950.

30. SWEET, W. H., and WEPSIC, J. G.: Treatment of pain by chronic electrical stimulation of large nerve fibers. Presented at meeting of the American Assoc. of Neurological Surgeons, Cleveland, Ohio, April 1969.

31. TOMASCH, J., and BRITTON, W. A.: On the individual variability of fibre composition in human peripheral nerves. *J Anat,* 90:337, 1956.

32. VON FREY, M.: Beitrage zur Sinnesphysiologie der Haut. III. Ber sachs. *Ges Wiss Math-Phys Cl,* 47:166, 1895.

33. WHITE, J. C., and SWEET, W. H.: *Pain: Its Mechanisms and Neurosurgical Control.* Springfield, Thomas, 1955.

Chapter 14

MUSCLE PAIN

Simon Rodbard*

CERTAIN preneuronal aspects of pain can be demonstrated readily in contracting muscle. This type of pain can be induced in less than a minute by repeatedly flexing the hand as rapidly as possible (7). A slight pain appears in the flexor muscles of the arm after twenty to thirty contractions. As the exercise continues for approximately another thirty contractions, the severity of the pain increases until it becomes intolerable, and the muscles seem so weak that they can no longer be contracted voluntarily. The pain appears even more quickly if a tourniquet obstructs blood flow into the arm.

Like other pain, this sensation so engages the attention of the subject that the search for relief becomes his primary activity. The severity of the pain will cause the patient to thrash about and exhibit great irritability if the tourniquet is not removed. Finally, he will project his strong feelings against nearby persons or objects.

An essentially similar type of muscle pain is observed commonly in the syndrome of intermittent claudication. In this phenomenon, the reduced caliber of the supplying arteries restricts blood flow into the contracting muscles of the leg. Relief is readily obtained by cessation of the exercise. Activity can be resumed following even a brief interval of rest, but the pain recurs after only a few contractions and walking may become limited to a brief series of steps followed by longer and longer necessary intervals of rest.

Angina pectoris is a similar pain-producing syndrome associated with myocardial contraction. Intestinal angina, which occurs in mesenteric artery stenosis, results in pain associated with a reduced blood supply to involuntary muscle. Control of the beating of the heart and of intestinal peristalsis is independent of the volitional mechanisms of the nervous system, and thus the contractions continue and the pain may persist or increase in intensity. In the case of angina pectoris the heart may be slowed by carotid sinus stimulation, or morphine or other powerful pain-obtunding drugs may be administered to give relief. A problem in evaluat-

* Aided by Grant HE 08721 from the National Heart Institute of the United States Public Health Services.

ing pain reported by the patient is that the complaint is subjective and not easily standardized.

Intolerable pain of muscle demands that the muscle must stop contracting despite such serious consequences as death. For example, if someone at a height is hanging onto a rope, muscle pain will become so severe that even though the individual is aware that release of the rope will result in his death, he nevertheless will be unable to maintain his hold. An animal pursued by a predator must stop when the exercising muscles become fatigued or painful. The remarkable prepotency of the muscle pain mechanism, which takes precedence over almost all other voluntary functions, indicates its importance in the chemistry of contraction. These properties of the pain mechanism render the phenomenon objective, and thus examination of factors that may contribute to the quantitative elucidation of the muscle pain mechanism becomes possible.

Despite the reality of the disturbances in muscle that lead to pain, especially in angina pectoris, the clinical evaluation of pain is remarkably difficult. The brain may evaluate impulses arising in the muscle in many different ways. Some patients with angina pectoris report crushing pain, others state that the sensation is a stabbing or burning discomfort, while still others have only a sense of fatigue.

Other muscle pains, usually of long duration, have been considered to result from spasm. For example, tension headaches have been attributed to spasm of the occipital muscles. Cramps represent another common form of muscle pain, but these symptoms have not been studied quantitatively. Trauma to muscles produces a boring, deep pain, but this is probably not dependent solely on a restricted blood supply. Finally, unaccustomed exercise generates a dull, aching muscle pain that can persist for several days even though the blood supply is presumably normal. This latter type of discomfort may be related to metabolic mechanisms involved in the induction of hypertrophy in the overloaded muscle. The pain is no longer noted when exercise becomes habitual.

Since the early work of Lewis (2) there has been consensus that during contraction muscle tissue produces a catabolite that induces the sensation of pain. Some aspects of this question can be investigated when there is no explicit interference with the blood flow to the muscle, as in arm exercise experiments in which no tourniquet is used.

Without Tourniquet

The author has examined the rate of development of pain when no tourniquet was applied on the arm of the experimental subjects. The subject contracted the muscles of the index finger to lift a 2.5 kg weight

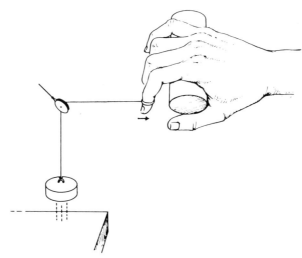

Figure 14-1. Method: Flexion of the index finger lifts weight a selected distance above the table.

3.5 cm above the surface of a table in a period of 0.5 second (Fig. 14-1). The rate of contraction affects the number of contractions that can be performed before pain brings exercise to a halt (Fig. 14-2).

Since the contraction phase of the cycle was constant in this series of tests the capacity to perform the exercise varied with a duration of muscle relaxation, when normal blood flow was probably taking place (Fig. 14-3). At forty contractions per minute the exercise could be continued fifteen minutes or longer without the development of significant pain. As the frequency of contraction increased and the intervals of muscle relaxation shortened, the number of contractions that could be performed before pain was evident declined.

These findings are consistent with the thesis that muscle contraction results in the accumulation of a catabolite that produces pain. When blood flow is adequate, as occurs during long relaxation intervals between successive contractions, the catabolite does not accumulate in sufficient quantities to initiate pain. At faster rates of contraction the relaxation interval and the resulting period for restoration of normal blood flow is inadequate to eliminate the pain-producing catabolite.

The effects of changes in arterial pressure on the tendency to cause pain were studied because the rate of blood flow appeared to be implicated in the elimination of pain. To do this we compared the number of contractions that could be performed when the arm was in a position horizontal to the body with the number performed when the arm was raised and supported at the elbow on an armrest. Nearly twice as many

contractions could be performed when the arm was in the horizontal posi-
ion than when it was upright (6).

The arterial pressure in the muscles of the forearm is reduced by
about 25 mm Hg when the arm is held upright. Under these circumstances the brachial arterial perfusion appears to be less effective in elim-
inating the pain factor from the exercising forearm muscles. It is possible
that an elevated arterial pressure would be expected to increase the per-

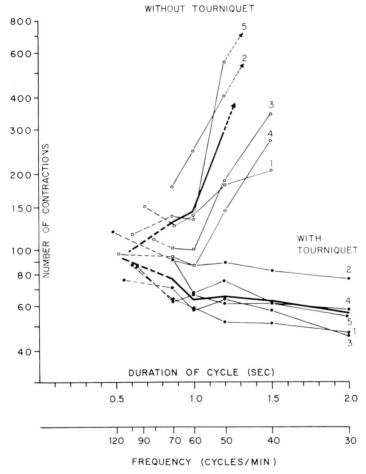

Figure 14-2. Duration of cycle (abscissa) plotted against the number of contractions performed (ordinate, logarithmic). The abscissa also gives the frequency in cycles/minute.
Data to the left of a rate of 70/min (----) were self-selected maximal rates. The number
of contractions performed with tourniquet is shown by —·—·. The number of contractions
performed without a tourniquet is shown by -o-o-. The heavy lines give the mean values
for each group. In the experiments without tourniquet, at long durations of the cycle,
the arrows represent the capacity to perform the exercise indefinitely.

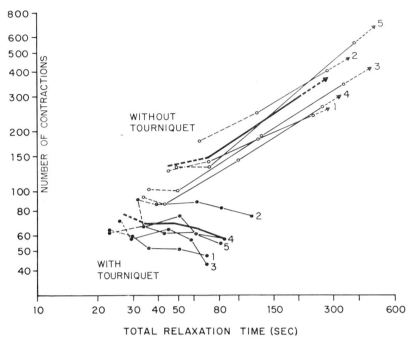

Figure 14-3. Number of contractions (ordinate, logarithmic) plotted against total relaxation time (abscissa, logarithmic). Conventions as in Figure 14-2.

fusion of the contracting muscle. Malinow *et al.* (3) have shown that arterial pressure tends to rise in intermittent claudication. Perhaps this increase is a means of compensation, which eliminates the pain factor.

With Tourniquet

In the foregoing experiments two opposing processes were apparently going on simultaneously. A pain-inducing catabolite was probably being produced during each contraction, and the flow of blood, especially during the interval of relaxation, operated in some way to eliminate this catabolite. Our data (5) indicate that the quantity of this noxious catabolite varies with the quantity of mechanical tension developed by the muscle.

Elimination of one of the two variables provides a more direct approach to the problem. We therefore eliminated the factor of blood flow by applying a tourniquet, consisting of a blood pressure cuff inflated to a suprasystolic pressure, to the upper arm (8) so that the rate of production of the pain-causing catabolite could be observed.

The number of times the index finger could lift the weight was sharply limited (Fig. 14-2), and intolerable pain occurred invariably within two minutes. As the duration of the contraction-relaxation cycle was prolonged, the number of contractions became minimal when the cycle was shortest. It appears that some factor, in addition to increased tension developed by the muscle, modifies the time when pain becomes evident. The results also indicate that the relaxed muscle does not detoxify nor eliminate the pain-producing catabolite.

Experiments in which the performance of the horizontal arm was compared with that of the elevated arm were repeated with blood flow obstructed by a tourniquet. The efficiency of the arm in the horizontal position was negated by the tourniquet.

It was then of interest to examine quantitative aspects of the production of the presumed pain-causing catabolite.

Muscle Tension

In these studies a tourniquet obstructed blood flow into the exercising arm. The subjects compressed the air in a rubber bulb to raise the mercury column 50, 100 or 200 mm for one second. The bulb was then

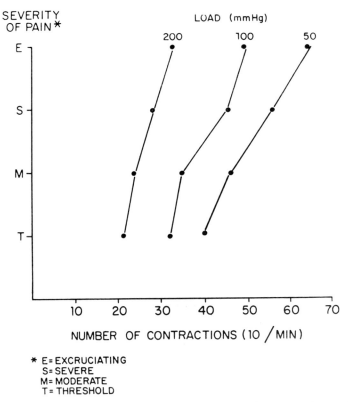

Figure 14-4. Relation of number of contractions performed at a rate of 10/min (abscissa) to the severity of pain (ordinate). Pain levels are T=Threshold, M=Moderate, S=Severe and E=Excruciating. Values are shown for work loads of 200, 100 or 50 mm Hg.

released. The grade of the pain was reported as threshold (T), moderate (M), severe (S) or excruciating (E), and the number of contractions for these grades of pain was recorded.

The data show an inverse relationship between the load and the number of contractions (Fig. 14-4).

The effect of the duration of contraction was studied by having the subject maintain the mercury column at the selected height for 1, 2, 4 or 5.5 seconds. The number of contractions decreased as the duration of contraction increased.

The data indicate that the severity of pain could be related to the product (P) of the number of contractions (C), the square root of the load (L) and the cube root of the duration (D) of each contraction:

$$P = C \cdot L^{0.5} \cdot D^{0.33} \text{ (Fig. 14-5)}.$$

Pain did not appear until P was approximately 300. The severity of

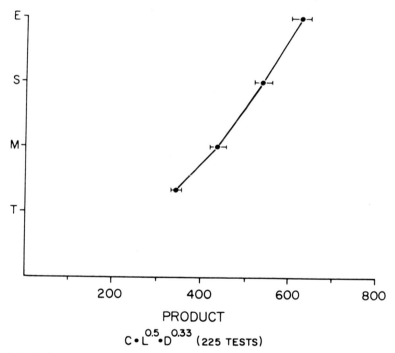

Figure 14-5. Relation of severity of pain to the product of the number of contractions (C), the square root of the load ($L^{0.5}$) and the cube root of the duration ($D^{0.33}$). Standard deviations for the product are shown for each level of severity of pain. Severity of pain as in Figure 14-4.

pain increased to moderate at 425, severe at 550 and excruciating at 670. The small standard deviation at each level indicates that the results are reproducible.

Data obtained on the total duration of a maintained contraction were comparable to those obtained when the contraction was of 5.5 seconds duration, with release for 0.5 second, and with immediate recontraction.

When the pain was reported to be excruciating, the blood pressure cuff was deflated and the pain was relieved instantly as blood flow was resumed.

The foregoing findings suggest that pain is related to the total tension developed during the contraction. The nonlinear effect of the duration of contraction may have been due to the fact that gripping movement is initiated by a limited set of available muscle bundles. When the grip is maintained, other muscle bundles contract and permit the previously contracted muscle bundles to relax. The similarity of the results obtained for gripping movements of 5.5 seconds duration and for maintained grips is consistent with the suggestion that the effects of duration are due to alternation of contractions of different muscle bundles. The product may vary with the square root of the load, perhaps because of the mechanical advantage of the tendons of the hand.

Metabolic Aspects

The development of pain could not be attributed to oxygen depletion in the tissues of the arm. Thus, obstruction of blood flow to the resting arm did not lead to the development of pain unless ischemia was maintained for more than ten minutes (Fig. 14-6). Further support for the thesis that the pain is not due to simple ischemia was obtained in findings that occlusion of the blood flow to the arm for ten or fifteen minutes had no significant effect on the number of contractions that could then be performed while the tourniquet remained in place. Occlusion of blood flow for twenty minutes, however, was associated with a reduction in the number of contractions. The pain under these conditions was associated with a discomfort that differed significantly in quality from the pain that was usually perceived after muscle contraction. This discomfort had a tingling component, perhaps from anoxia or ischemia of nerve bundles compressed by the tourniquet.

The pain factor is probably not dependent on the amount of oxygen in the blood delivered to the muscles. The contractions of subjects were observed while in a compression chamber breathing pure oxygen at three atmospheres of pressure (5). This is fifteen times the partial pressure of oxygen in air at sea level. High oxygen concentrations in the air that is

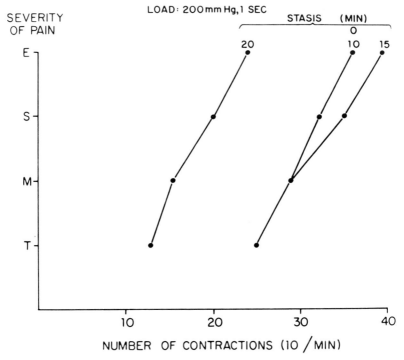

Figure 14-6. Effect of preliminary vascular stasis for periods of 10, 15 and 20 min on the subsequent number of contractions that produce varying levels of pain. Severity of pain as in Figure 14-4. The work load was 200 mm Hg maintained for 1 sec. Contractions were performed at a rate of 10/min.

breathed, and presumably in the tissues, has no effect on the number of contractions that can be performed.

The factor causing pain cannot be lactic acid. Neither lactic acid nor other products of the Kreb's cycle appear in the muscle or blood of patients with McArdle's disease, who have a deficiency of the phosphorylase that converts muscle glycogen to lactic acid. Ischemic muscle exercise in such patients results in pain that appears to be even more severe than in normal individuals (4).

Washout Experiments

The rate at which the pain-causing substance might be eliminated by the blood stream was observed. In this series of experiments, the subject wearing a tourniquet performed hand gripping movements until he could no longer withstand the pain or until he could no longer contract the fist because of fatigue (1). Pain was relieved when the blood pressure cuff was deflated. The pressure cuff was then reinflated to stop the blood flow to determine whether all the catabolite had been eliminated. A two-second interval of blood flow brought about complete apparent relief of the pain, but the number of gripping movements then achieved was only about one-fourth that in the initial test (Fig. 14-7). Thus, even though the pain has been relieved, something remains in the muscle that induces pain. When the interval of blood flow was extended to eight seconds before reapplication of the cuff and reinstitution of the exercise, the number of contractions increased to 40 percent of the initial number. After sixty-four seconds, about 75 percent as many contractions could be performed as in the initial test. These data appeared to follow a logarithmic decay curve, and extrapolation suggests that complete recovery of the capacity to perform exercise would be regained only after about ten minutes of unimpeded blood flow. Blood flow for one minute should have been adequate to restore preexercise conditions if the pain were due to lack of oxygen or to the washout of a highly diffusible substance. The failure of recovery in this interval indicates that the elimination of the agent responsible for pain depends on other time-limited mechanisms.

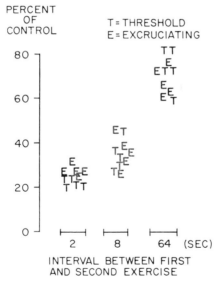

Figure 14-7. Effect of restoration of blood flow on recovery from pain. The control number of gripping contractions prior to threshold pain (T) and excruciating pain (E) in five trials at eighty per minute in each of four subjects was set at 100%. The cuff pressure was then dropped to atmospheric values for 2, 8 or 64 sec, following which the cuff was reinflated and the exercise repeated. The number of contractions before pain and before excruciating pain during the second exercise is shown as percent of that subject's control value. Recovery averages 20% after 2 sec of resumption of blood flow, about 35% after 8 seconds and about 70% after 64 seconds.

Such a limitation may be ascribed to slow diffusion of the pain-causing catabolite. The mechanism would differ markedly from that responsible for the rapid elimination of the sensation of pain by even the brief interval of two seconds of blood flow.

These findings support the thesis that some substance persists in the muscle despite a relatively long period (64 seconds) of blood flow and metabolic exchange. This persistence may be attributed to the slow diffusion of a large molecule from its site of production in the muscle fiber to an extracellular locus from which it can be eliminated, perhaps by being washed away.

Diffusion

Molecules of catabolite that remain in the muscle fibers continue to diffuse slowly into the extracellular fluid and into the vicinity of pain-responsive fibers. A slow rate of diffusion would require many minutes for the complete elimination of the pain-producing catabolite from the tissue. This concept of diffusion is supported by unpublished experiments in which intolerable pain was induced by exercise of the arm with a tourniquet, after which the normal flow of blood was restored for four seconds. As expected, the pain was relieved completely. The tourniquet was then replaced, but the arm remained at rest. Pain gradually returned and became progressively more severe despite the fact that no new catabolite was being produced by the resting arm.

No Summation of Pain

In other studies we have found that pain in muscle does not summate. When both hands are exercised simultaneously while a tourniquet is present on both arms, the number of contractions of each arm is approximately equal to that when only one arm is used. Only the most severe pain is noted; the other pains are ignored.

Mechanism

The findings in this report are consistent with the hypothesis that contracting muscle produces a catabolite that generates pain in that site. The production of pain-causing catabolite varies with the total tension developed, as indicated by the number of contractions, the load and the duration of the contraction.

Factors involved in the production of pain in ischemic muscle are summarized in Figure 14-8. This is a diagram illustrating a block of muscle tissue with a capillary that carries blood through the tissue.

Contraction of muscle is associated with the production of pain-causing catabolites inside muscle fibers. These catabolites diffuse slowly across the fiber membranes to enter the extracellular fluid of the tissues. The catabolites have no effect when their concentration in tissue fluids that bathe nociceptor fibers is less than half that required to produce excruciating pain. As the concentration of the catabolite in the vicinity of the nociceptor increases, either because of muscle contraction or because of a decreased rate of blood perfusion, the nociceptor is stimulated and impulses are transmitted to the central nervous system. The brain interprets these neural impulses as pain or fatigue.

The initiating event is thus preneural, arising in the metabolic activity of muscular contraction. A certain concentration of this material produces nerve impulses that the brain interprets as threshold or mild pain. About twice this threshold quantity produces intolerable pain. The sensation of pain is eliminated almost instantaneously with the onset of blood flow,

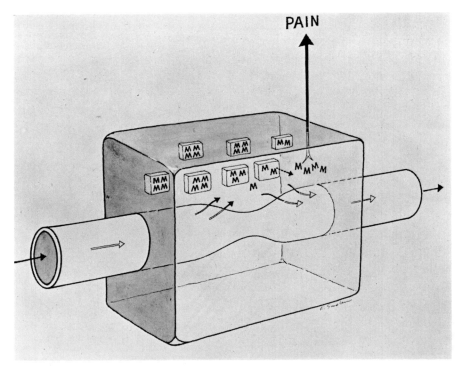

Figure 14-8. Concept of diffusion. Blood flow (arrow at left) through the capillary (central tube) is associated with ultrafiltration of fluid into the extracellular space (curved arrows leading out of capillary) and return of fluid via the downstream end of the capillary (curved arrows leading into vessel). Muscle cells (rectangles) produce end-products of metabolites (M) on contraction. These diffuse slowly out of the cells (dotted arrow). Accumulation of a threshold quantity of these catabolites at nociceptor nerve endings generates impulses which are interpreted by the central nervous system as pain.

presumably because the catabolite has been metabolized, washed away
or otherwise eliminated from tissue fluids.

Overview

Muscle contraction produces a substance that reduces the capacity of
the individual to continue to exercise. That this is not due to the ex-
haustion of materials that are necessary for the contractile process is indicated by the fact that muscles that have become "fatigued" by exercising to the point at which volitional contraction seems to be impossible
can still contract vigorously if the muscle is stimulated directly (6). This
suggests that the pain is not due to a deficiency, but to an excess of an
end-product of the contractile process. The end-product associated with
the pain process apparently cannot be metabolized or otherwise detoxified
in the muscle—it must be eliminated by the flowing blood.

If the catabolite is an end-product of muscle contraction, why is it not
simply an innocuous material that may be transported at the convenience
of local mechanisms, rather than being a material that can and does
threaten life? We must assume that the pain-causing substance is a highly
toxic material which can produce serious harm to the contractile ma-
chinery in which it is formed. In addition, it must be a necessary part of
the contractile mechanism. It is likely that minuscule quantities of the
material produce highly potent effects.

Why should muscle contraction, a key process in survival, be hobbled
by the toxic action of some product of the contraction itself? We may
speculate that the diffusion of relatively large toxic materials posed no
problems to the tiny organisms in which the mechanisms of contraction
first evolved. The subsequent incorporation of huge numbers of contractile units in the muscle cell then introduced problems of diffusion and
elimination of catabolites generated during contraction.

An adequate vascular bed can produce a stream of blood flow and,
perhaps of equal importance, mass transport of extracapillary fluid to
eliminate the pain catabolite. Failure of blood flow because of inadequate
perfusion pressure or because of vascular narrowing may permit the local
accumulation of intolerable concentrations of the catabolite.

Why does the nervous system not ignore the presence of the pain-producing catabolite? We may assume, on general biological grounds, that it
cannot, since local accumulation of this material would be highly toxic
to the tissues.

It appears, then, that a toxic material of significant molecular weight is
produced in the course of muscle contraction. The blood stream neu-
tralizes or transports this material away from the muscle cells. Attempts

to isolate this substance may provide means for the further elucidation of elements of the contractile process, the mechanism of stimulation of nociceptive nerve fibers, the adequate inhibition of the toxicity of the substance and the clarification of other problems related to pain.

SUMMARY

Experiments on the production of pain in ischemic exercising muscle are discussed briefly. The development of contractile tension is associated with the production in the muscle fiber of a diffusible catabolite that can stimulate pain fibers. The severity of pain varied with the product of the number of contractions, the square root of the load and the cube root of the duration of contraction. About half of the quantity of the catabolite that causes excruciating pain is necessary to produce a threshold or slight pain. The catabolite is probably a fairly large molecule that diffuses slowly out of its site of production in the muscle fiber. It probably is not lactic acid or carbon dioxide, and it is not due to oxygen deficiency. Ischemia produced by occlusion of blood supply without contraction does not augment or produce muscle pain. The most severe pain dominates the sensorium; there is no summation of simultaneous, separate pains. This pain mechanism causes the individual to seek immediate relief from pain.

REFERENCES

1. HORISBERGER, B., and RODBARD, S.: Relation between pain and fatigue in contracting ischemic muscle. *Amer J Cardiol*, 8:481, 1961.
2. LEWIS, T.: *Pain*. New York, Macmillan, 1942.
3. MALINOW, M. R.; MOIA, B.; OTERO, E., and ROSENBAUM, M.: The occurrence of paroxysmal hypertension in patients with intermittent claudication. *Amer Heart J.* 38:702, 1949.
4. MCARDLE, B.: Myopathy due to defect in muscle glycogen breakdown. *Clin Sci*, 10:13. 1951.
5. PARK, S. R., and RODBARD, S.: Effect of load and duration of tension on pain induced by muscular contraction. *Amer J Physiol*, 203:735, 1962.
6. RODBARD, S.: Unpublished data.
7. RODBARD, S., and PRAGAY, E. B.: Contraction frequency, blood supply, and muscle pain. *J Applied Physiol*, 24:142, 1968.
8. ZAK, E.: Uber den Gefassskrampf bei intermittierendem Hinken und uber gewisse Kapillomotorische Erscheinungen. *Wien Z Inn Med*, 2:405, 1921.

Chapter 15

SOME CURRENT VIEWS ON THE
NEUROPHYSIOLOGY OF PAIN

Kenneth L. Casey*

VARIOUS and often opposing hypotheses about the neural mechanisms of the sensation of pain have developed in parallel throughout the history of the neurological sciences. Thus, in a sense, there may be little in the more recent hypotheses that is really "new" from the conceptual point of view. Nonetheless, the validity of one conceptual model or another has rested upon the emergence of the new experimental or clinical findings, so that the sorting out and modification of old ideas may give the impression of new theoretical concepts being developed. With this in mind, we can examine the development of some of the more recent views regarding neural mechanisms in pain sensation.

One of the major concepts forming the basis for many hypotheses about mechanisms of pain is that of functional localization within the nervous system. On the basis of the anatomical and physiological organization of other sensory systems, it has seemed reasonable to expect that pain would have its distinct central pathways and peripheral receptors. Among the somatic sensations, pain has seemed sufficiently unique to warrant this anatomical distinction. The problem arises in the specificity with which structure and function can be correlated.

The contention of von Frey in 1895 (21), that free nerve endings are "pain receptors" and that excitation of these endings or receptors resulted in pain sensation gained widespread acceptance. Subsequent physiological (15) and psychophysiological (23) experiments implicated finely myelinated and unmyelinated fibers as subserving "epicritic" and "protopathic" pain mechanisms. However, current anatomical (50) and psychological (30) evidence indicates that free nerve endings must function as receptors for many other forms of somatic sensation and are not exclusively "pain receptors." Furthermore, recent physiological studies (19, 27, 28) have shown that the small diameter afferents do not, as a group, respond only to intense stimuli. Indeed, the majority of those studied are quite sensitive to thermal or mechanical stimuli, and many are sensi-

* Grant NB-06588 from the National Institute of Neurological Diseases and Stroke has supported some of the original work referred to in this article. The author is greatly indebted to to Dr. Ronald Melzack for many helpful and informative discussions.

tive to both forms of energy (24). Within the population of unmyelinated and, in particular, finely myelinated fibers, however, is a group of cutaneous afferents responding only to intense mechanical (7) or thermal (24) stimuli. The nociceptive function of some small-diameter afferents is further suggested by clinical and human neurophysiological studies (16, 48) showing that pain sensation is elicited only in conjunction with fine fiber activity. The small-diameter afferents involved may not all share the characteristics of high threshold to physiologic stimuli, for in certain pathological conditions gentle stimuli produce painful or unpleasant sensations. Noordenbos (41) has reported an increase in the proportion of fine cutaneous fibers in herpetic neuropathy, but whether or not these pathologic conditions alter the functional effect of large-diameter fibers remains to be determined. The existence of hyperpathic or hyperalgesic phenomena does, however, indicate that the physiologically determined sensitivity of a primary cutaneous afferent bears no necessary relationship to its participation in the production of the sensation of pain.

At present, then, there would seem to be a reasonably satisfying functional-structural correlation at the peripheral nerve level: fine cutaneous afferent activity appears to be a necessary condition for pain sensation. How do these fibers produce this unique effect and what are the CNS pathways and mechanisms involved? One view of functional localization would suggest a well-defined set of central neurons and pathways activated exclusively by small-diameter afferents. But the majority of these primary afferents are sensitive to innocuous and normally nonpainful stimuli; clearly, additional modifications of this hypothesis would be required. One answer to these and related problems has been essentially to abandon the concept of functional localization so far as pain is concerned and to emphasize the importance of the temporal pattern of the afferent input (51). The arguments concerning "pattern" and "specificity" theories of cutaneous sensory mechanisms have been considered in detail by Melzack and Wall (34) and need no further elaboration here. The importance of spatial and temporal mechanisms of coding is well established for the nervous system; elements of both are required in considering the neuroanatomical and neurophysiological basis for pain.

A dorsal horn "gate" mechanism, proposed by Melzack and Wall (35) as part of the neural mechanism for pain, has offered another way of looking at the unique effects of fine afferent fibers. The gate mechanism is based on the physiological experiments of Mendell and Wall (37), who showed that small-diameter fiber volleys potentiate ventral root reflexes evoked by large fiber volleys. This potentiation was considered to reflect the release of primary afferent terminals from a tonic presynaptic inhibition by substantia gelatinosa cells. Recording the slow potential at the dorsal root suggested that large cutaneous afferents, acting via the substantia gelatinosa, *depolarize* the intramedullary afferent terminals and thus *decrease* the effectiveness of excitatory synapses, while small-diameter fibers oppose this effect. The firing frequency of some spinal cord neurons would, then, depend on the relative amounts of large or small fiber input; intramedullary and supraspinal connections of these cells would reflect this sensitivity to small-diameter cutaneous afferents. This kind of interaction mechanism could also explain the decrease in pain brought about by electrical stimulation of the dorsal columns (46) or large cutaneous afferents (49) without postulating complex temporal codes or specialized pain pathways. The physiological basis for the gate hypothesis, however, has been seriously questioned. Franz and Iggo (20) did not find evidence of an opposing presynaptic action of large and small fibers. Furthermore, their results indicated that the reflex-potentiating effect of small fiber volleys could be explained by spatial and temporal summation of excitatory inputs at a common neuron pool. At present, then, it would appear that much remains to be done before the mechanism of the effects of small fibers is satisfactorily understood at the neurophysiological level.

Whatever the mechanism, there is now substantial evidence that small cutaneous afferents can profoundly influence the activity of some central neurons. C fiber volleys have been shown to increase the frequency and duration of discharge of spinal neurons receiving somatic input (36). Earlier studies (17, 18) have revealed similar effects on evoked potential and multiple unit discharge in the mesencephalic reticular formation. Stimulation of finely myelinated (A delta) fibers also greatly increases the poststimulus response of neurons in the mesencephalic (5) and medial medullary (11) reticular formation, a finding of particular relevance to pain mechanisms, since studies on man have shown that pain is first reported when this fiber population is activated (18). Experiments recently completed in the laboratory (11) show that in the unanesthetized, decerebrate and decerebellate cat, the majority of responsive cells in the medial bulboreticular formation (n. gigantocellularis of Olzewski) are excited only by intense mechanical stimuli over some part of their receptive field and are driven maximally only when the afferent volley includes A delta fibers. Since stimulation of the larger-diameter A fibers had a small but definite excitatory effect on many of these neurons, anodal polarization of cutaneous nerve was used (13) to block the larger fibers and reveal the differential effect of finely myelinated afferents.

Neurons responding maximally only to intense stimuli have been recorded in other areas of the reticular formation (8), spinal cord (29).

thalamus (43, 44) and cortex (9). In the awake, partially restrained squirrel monkey, medial and posterolateral thalamic units responsive to innocuous stimuli showed prolonged and more intense responses to stimuli that consistently produced withdrawal of the stimulated limb (10). The effect of fine afferent fiber stimulation, however, has not been determined in most of these studies.

Taken together, the physiological observations to date would suggest a differentially responding population that would trigger the sensation of pain and response when its activity reached a certain critical level. As Becker has observed (5), the "summation" theory of pain is not new, but has not received much attention in recent years. However, combined electrophysiological and behavioral experiments relevant to this concept are currently underway in this laboratory. Some medial bulboreticular units in the cat have been observed to respond to electrical cutaneous nerve stimuli well below the threshold for eliciting a trained escape response (barrier crossing), but show progressive increases in poststimulus discharge as the stimulus approaches the behavioral escape threshold. Electrical stimulation of this same bulboreticular area will elicit escape responses in the trained cat or can be used as unconditioned stimuli in the naive animal.

Certain brain stem reticular formation neurons, then, do appear to participate in pain mechanisms. But what relation could their activity have to pain phenomena? Pain, as we have suggested elsewhere, consists of at least two dimensions: discriminative and motivational. The reticular formation and other extralemniscal pathways do not have the physiological properties that indicate a role in fine spatial and temporal localization or in the recognition of details about the physical nature of the stimulus (2). These discriminative functions are more likely to be performed via the classical lemniscal system, which includes the dorsal column, dorsolateral and neospinothalamic (32) pathways. Neurons in the reticular formation, however, form part of a brain stem region intimately connected with the limbic system (31, 45). Spinoreticular fibers ascending in the anterolateral quadrant of the spinal cord project to the medial brain stem reticular formation and the midbrain central gray (33). This "limbic midbrain area" (38) projects diffusely to the adjacent reticular formation, is connected reciprocally with the hypothalamus via Schutz' fasciculus, forms a significant part of the input to medial and intralaminar thalamic nuclei and receives projections from the frontal granular cortex (39, 40). This brain stem region shares with limbic forebrain structures the property of relatively direct hypothalamic connections. The limbic system is now known to play a major role in basic, motivational be-

havioral mechanisms, and it is well established that stimulation or ablation of certain limbic system structures profoundly influences aversive
drives or pain-related behavior. As we have indicated elsewhere (12, 14),
the evidence suggests that limbic structures, although playing a role in
many other functions (45), provide a neural basis for the aversive drive
and affect comprising the motivational dimension of pain. Since the activity of some brain stem reticular neurons is influenced by intense natural somatic stimuli and fine afferent fiber input and, on stimulation and
recording, appears to be associated with escape behavior, there is reason
to suggest that the aversive aspect of pain is determined, at least in part,
by the level of activity within this neural population.

Pain, however, is not exclusively influenced by the presence or absence
of intense somatic stimuli or fine afferent fiber input. A number of investigators (4, 6, 42) have shown that pain is affected profoundly by en-
vironmental and psychological factors that must involve "higher" central
processes. Many forebrain structures can influence the activity of ascending pathways in the spinal cord and reticular formation. Descending influences from the cortex (3) and reticular formation (26) act at dorsal
horn levels to modify the synaptic effectiveness of primary afferent fibers
and regulate the amount of ascending activity (22). Neocortical (1) and
limbic forebrain areas (25) also influence the activity in brainstem reticular formation. The anatomical and physiological evidence (12) leaves
little doubt that complex psychological processes represented in the function of higher levels of the nervous system can influence transfer of information at many levels. The concept of "central control" has been incorporated in the "gate" hypothesis (35), in which it was suggested that
descending influences could be triggered by the rapidly conducting fibers
of the lemniscal system. However activated, these central descending influences comprise an additional determinant of pain that is no less important than the intensity of somatic input or the presence of fine afferent fiber activity.

Both basic research and clinical observation, then, have contributed to
current concepts about the neural mechanisms of pain. As more information becomes available, these concepts will certainly change. For the present, however, it would appear that the long-standing association between
fine afferent fiber activity and sensation of pain is supported. Details regarding the mechanisms of the action of fine fibers are currently the
subject of much controversy, but there is little doubt as to their importance in influencing the activity of central cells, particularly those in certain regions of the reticular formation. There is evidence that some of
these reticular formation neurons play an important role in pain mech-

anisms and their potential anatomical association with the limbic system and lack of fine somatotopic organization suggest a motivational rather than a discriminative function. Other members of this same population may influence motor response patterns related to nociception by way of well-known reticulospinal projections (47, 52). In any case, the level of activity of some of these reticular cells may prove to be one of the important determinants of pain. Finally, it is important to recognize the influence of "higher" central nervous system structures on the afferent and ascending systems that may be a part of the pain mechanism. Pain can be regarded as somewhat unique in having both motivational and discriminative aspects as critical determinants; as in other sensory systems, however, the influence of descending pathways may be equally critical. The neural mechanism of pain must include all of these determinants, and pain cannot be ascribed solely to any one of them.

REFERENCES

1. Adey, W. R.; Segundo, J. P., and Livingston, R. B.: Corticofugal influences on intrinsic brain stem conduction in cat and monkey. *J Neurophysiol*, 20:1, 1957.

2. Albe-Fessard, D.: Organization of Somatic Central Projections. In Neff, W. D. (Ed.): *Contributions to Sensory Physiology*. New York, Academic, 1967, vol. 2.

3. Anderson, P.; Eccles, J. C., and Sears, T. A.: Cortically evoked depolarization of primary afferent fibers in the spinal cord. *J Neurophysiol*, 27:63, 1964.

4. Barber, T. X.: Toward a theory of pain: Relief of chronic pain by prefrontal leucotomy, opiates, placebos, and hypnosis. *Psychol Bull*, 56:430, 1959.

5. Becker, D. P.; Gluck, H.; Mulsen, F. E., and Jane, J. A.: An inquiry into the neurophysiological basis for pain. *J Neurosurg*, 30:1, 1969.

6. Beecher, H. K.: *Measurement of Subjective Responses*. New York, Oxford U.P., 1959.

7. Burgess, P. R., and Perl, E. R.: Myelinated afferent fibers responding specifically to noxious stimulation of the skin. *J Physiol*, 190:541, 1967.

8. Burton, H.: Somatic sensory properties of caudal bulbar reticular neurons in the cat (felis domestica). *Brain Res*, 11:357, 1968.

9. Carreras, M., and Anderson, S. A.: Functional properties of neurons of the anterior ectosylvian gyrus of the cat. *J Neurophysiol*, 26:100, 1963.

10. Casey, K. L.: Nociceptive mechanisms in the thalamus of awake squirrel monkey. *J Neurophysiol*, 29:727, 1966.

11. Casey, K. L.: Somatic stimuli, spinal pathways, and size of cutaneous fibers influencing unit activity in the medial medullary reticular formation. *Exp Neurol*, 25:35-56, 1969.

12. Casey, K. L.: Toward a neurophysiology of pain. *Headache*, 9:141, 1969.

13. Casey, K. L., and Blick, M.: Observations on anodal polarization of cutaneous nerve. *Brain Res*, 13:155, 1969.

14. Casey, K. L., and Melzack, R.: Neural mechanisms of pain: a conceptual model. In: Way, E. Leong (Ed.): *New Concepts in Pain and Its Clinical Management*. Philadelphia, Davis, 1967.

15. CLARK, D.; HUGHES, J., and GASSER, H. S.: Afferent function in the group of nerve fibers of slowest conduction velocity. *Amer J Physiol*, 114:69, 1935.

16. COLLINS, W. F.; NULSEN, F. E., and RANDT, C. T.: Relation of peripheral nerve fiber size and sensation in man. *Arch Neurol (Chicago)*, 3:381, 1960.

17. COLLINS, W. F., and O'LEARY, J. L.: Study of a somatic evoked response of midbrain reticular substance. *Electroenceph Clin Neurophysiol*, 6:619, 1954.

18. COLLINS, W. F., and RANDT, C. T.: Midbrain evoked responses relating to peripheral unmyelinated or "C" fibers in cat. *J Neurophysiol*, 23:47, 1960.

19. DOUGLAS, W. W., and RITCHIE, J. M.: Non-medullated fibers in the saphenous nerve which signal touch. *J Physiol (London)*, 139:385, 1957.

20. FRANZ, D. N., and IGGO, A.: Dorsal root potentials and ventral root reflexes evoked by nonmyelated fibers. *Science*, 162:1140, 1968.

21. FREY, M. VON.: Beitrage zur Sinnesphysiologie der Haut. *Ber d kgl sachs Ges d Wiss Math-Phys Kl*, 47:181, 1895.

22. HAGBARTH, K. E., and FEX, J.: Centrifugal influences on single unit activity in spinal sensory paths. *J Neurophysiol*, 22:321, 1959.

23. HEINBECKER, P.; BISHOP, G. H., and O'LEARY, J.: Pain and touch fibers in peripheral nerves. *Arch Neurol (Chicago)*, 29:771, 1933.

24. HENSEL, H.; IGGO, A., and WITT, I.: A quantitative study of sensitive cutaneous thermoreceptors with C afferent fibres. *J Physiol (London)*, 153:113, 1960.

25. HERNANDEZ-PEON, R., and HAGBARTH, K. E.: Interaction between afferent and cortically induced reticular responses. *J Neurophysiol*, 18:43, 1955.

26. HOLMQVIST, R.; LUNDBERG, A., and OSCARSSON, O.: Supraspinal inhibitory control of transmission to three ascending spinal pathways influenced by the flexion reflex afferents. *Arch Ital Biol*, 98:60, 1960.

27. HUNT, C. C., and McINTYRE, A. K.: An analysis of fibre diameter and receptor characteristics of myelinated cutaneous afferent fibres in cat. *J Physiol (London)*, 153:99, 1960.

28. IGGO, A.: Cutaneous mechanoreceptors with afferent C fibers. *J Physiol (London)*, 152:337, 1960.

29. KOLMODIN, G. M., and SKOGLUND, C. R.: Analysis of spinal interneurons activated by tactile and nociceptive stimulation. *Acta Physiol Scand*, 50:337, 1960.

30. LELE, P. P., and WEDDELL, G.: Sensory nerves in the cornea and cutaneous sensibility. *Exp Neurol*, 1:334, 1959.

31. MACLEAN, P. D.: Psychosomatic disease and the "visceral brain." Recent developments bearing on the Papez theory of emotion. *Psychosom Med*, 11:338, 1949.

32. MEHLER, W. R.: The mammalian "pain tract" in phylogeny. *Anat Rec*, 127:332, 1957.

33. MEHLER, W. R.; FEFERMAN, M. E., and NAUTA, W. J. H.: Ascending axon degeneration following antero-lateral cordotomy. An experimental study in the monkey. *Brain*, 83:718, 1960.

34. MELZACK, R., and WALL, P. D.: On the nature of cutaneous sensory mechanisms. *Brain*, 85:331, 1962.

35. MELZACK, R., and WALL, P. D.: Pain mechanisms: A new theory. *Science*, 150:971, 1965.

36. MENDELL, L. M.: Physiological properties of unmyelinated fiber projection to the spinal cord. *Exp Neurol*, 16:316, 1966.

37. MENDELL, L. M., and WALL, P. D.: Presynaptic hyperpolarization: A role for fine afferent fibres. *J. Physiol (London)*, 172:274, 1964.

38. NAUTA, W. J. H.: Hippocampal projections and related neural pathways to the midbrain in the cat. *Brain*, 81:319, 1958.
39. NAUTA, W. J. H.: Some efferent connections of the prefrontal cortex in the monkey. In Warren, J. M., and Akert, K. (Eds.): *The Frontal Granular Cortex and Behavior*. New York, McGraw, 1964.
40. NEWMAN, P. P., and WOLSTENCROFT, J. H.: Medullary responses to stimulation of orbital cortex. *J Neurophysiol*, 22:516, 1959.
41. NOORDENBOS, W.: *Pain*. Amsterdam, Elsevier, 1959.
42. PAVLOV, I. P.: *Lectures on Conditioned Reflexes*. New York, Int. Pubs., 1928.
43. PERL, E. R., and WHITLOCK, D. G.: Somatic stimuli exciting spinothalamic projections to thalamic neurons in cat and monkey. *Exp Neurol*, 3:256, 1961.
44. POGGIO, G. F., and MOUNTCASTLE, V. B.: A study of the functional contributions of the lemniscal and spinothalamic systems to somatic sensibility. *Bull Hopkins Hosp*, 106:266, 1960.
45. PRIBRAM, K. H., and KRUGER, L.: Functions of the "olfactory brain." *Ann NY Acad Sci*, 58:109, 1964.
46. SHEALY, C. N.; MORTIMER, J. T., and RESWICK, J. B.: Electrical inhibition of pain by stimulation of the dorsal columns: Preliminary clinical report. *Anesth Analg (Cleveland)*, 46:489, 1967.
47. SPRAGUE, J. M., and CHAMBERS, W. W.: Control of posture by reticular formation and cerebellum in the intact, anesthetized and unanesthetized and in the decerebrated cat. *Amer J Physiol*, 176:52, 1954.
48. SWANSON, A. G.; BUCHAN, G. C., and ALVORD, E. C.: Anatomic changes in congenital insensitivity to pain. *Arch Neurol (Chicago)*, 12:12, 1965.
49. WALL, P. D., and SWEET, W. H.: Temporary abolition of pain in man. *Science*, 155:108, 1967.
50. WEDDELL, G.; PALMER, E., and PALLIE, W.: Nerve endings in mammalian skin. *Biol Rev*, 30:159, 1955.
51. WEDDELL, G., and MILLER, S.: Cutaneous sensibility. *Ann Rev Physiol*, 24:199, 1962.
52. WOLSTENCROFT, J. H.: Reticulospinal neurones. *J Physiol (London)*, 174:91, 1964.

Chapter 16

STRATEGIES AND TACTICS IN THE TREATMENT OF PATIENTS WITH PAIN

RICHARD A. STERNBACH

IN this paper I will discuss, primarily, ways of *thinking about* pain. The purpose is to show that the way we think about pain tends to lock us into patterns of treatment (and research) that are not as productive or useful as they might be. Of course, most pain patterns are well understood and the sufferers can well be treated; but around the edges of these patterns now are numerous cases of "intractable," "paradoxical" and "recurrent" pain which baffle and annoy us. I hope to suggest alternative ways of thinking about pain which may provide us with more flexibility in dealing with such patients.

The basic problem seems to be with our language; we use words to describe something, like "pain," and then are unable to free ourselves from the words to come up with a fresh description. Let me illustrate this with a crude story, which I hope will provide enough of a jolt to let you see that the use of our language can be silly indeed.

When I was in the Army I became friends with a full-blooded Cherokee named Wolfchief. One drunken night we had a small ceremony and became "blood-brothers." In the quiet conversation that followed, Wolfchief confessed that there were some things about the white man that puzzled him. "You palefaces sure talk funny," he said. "For instance, you say you're going to *take* a shit; the Indian says he's going to *leave* one." I had to agree that he had a point.

Now let us look at the ways we have of thinking about pain, which seem to me to be similarly silly. In Figure 16-1 are listed some of the current views of pain. Your choice of what pain *is* will depend, mostly, upon your profession. If you are an experimental psychologist, you may prefer the traditional view that pain is a basic, elementary sensation, like sight or hearing; or you may accept the view that it is a complex perception influenced by past experiences, current needs, etc. Psychiatrists, on the other hand, usually treat pain as though it were an affect or emotion, like anger or depression or anxiety; or, if they have a traditional psychoanalytic orientation, they may emphasize the internal psychic conflict which results in pain as a symptom.

If you are a neurologist or neurosurgeon, it is fairly certain that you

CURRENT WAYS OF VIEWING PAIN

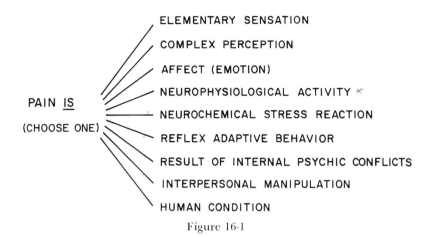

PAIN IS

(CHOOSE ONE)

ELEMENTARY SENSATION

COMPLEX PERCEPTION

AFFECT (EMOTION)

NEUROPHYSIOLOGICAL ACTIVITY

NEUROCHEMICAL STRESS REACTION

REFLEX ADAPTIVE BEHAVIOR

RESULT OF INTERNAL PSYCHIC CONFLICTS

INTERPERSONAL MANIPULATION

HUMAN CONDITION

Figure 16-1

think of pain as a pattern of neurophysiological activity, involving certain pathways and structures, or you may emphasize the importance of local chemical reactions to trauma. On the other hand, followers of recent developments in psychiatry and clinical psychology may choose the existentialist view, which has a long religious and philosophical tradition, that pain is the essence of the human condition; in pain we are supremely alone and thrown back onto ourselves, yet through pain we are linked to the rest of suffering humanity. Or we may focus on the interpersonal aspects of pain, seeing pain as a "game" through which we relate to others in a manipulative way. The biologist, of course, would emphasize the survival value of pain, seeing it as a reflexive adaptive process that functions to avoid trauma and death.

Now all these approaches to our views of pain are reasonable and, furthermore, have data to support them. The question arises, Which is the *correct* view? Surely one of these must be superior to the others. In this conference, most of us would probably prefer to put our money on the neurophysiological approach as the ultimate winner. After all, we have years of training invested in it, and our income depends on it; we have a vested interest. But can we make use of the other definitions as well, even though they seem contradictory? They are not "wrong," really, yet how can pain be all these many things?

In Figure 16-2, a relativistic definition is proposed, which I think may be of value in understanding pain. It emphasizes that the word "pain" is an abstraction that we use to refer to many different phenomena. One class of these phenomena includes a wide variety of subjective *experi-*

A RELATIVISTIC DEFINITION OF PAIN

"PAIN" IS AN ABSTRACT CONCEPT WHICH AN OBSERVER MAY USE TO DESCRIBE
(1) A PERSONAL, PRIVATE SENSATION OF HURT;
(2) A HARMFUL STIMULUS WHICH SIGNALS CURRENT OR IMPENDING TISSUE
    DAMAGE;
(3) A PATTERN OF RESPONSES WHICH OPERATE TO PROTECT THE ORGANISM
    FROM HARM.

Figure 16-2

ences, including the different sensations of stinging, aching, burning, stabbing hurts, etc. These are private experiences that are not directly available to clinical or experimental observation, but the word "pain" is used to refer to these collective experiences.

We also use the word "pain" to refer to the variety of observable noxious *stimuli* that are partly correlated with the subjective experiences: the heat, the cold, the pressure, the acids and the other physical traumata which result in actual or incipient tissue damage. We say, *"That* hurts," referring to such stimuli.

Finally we also use the word "pain" to refer to the variety of observable *responses:* escape and avoidance behaviors, physiological reactions, neurochemical stress responses, verbalizations, etc. These are all the responses, from the level of the molecular to the level of gross overt behavior, that are elicited by pain stimuli, but which are only partially correlated with the stimuli and with the subjective experiences.

Since "pain" may refer to any of these phenomena, it is clear that it is an abstract concept. Furthermore, since tradition and usage justify such multiple meanings of the word, the observer's choice of how he will use the term is simply that—a choice that best suits his purposes, and thus this definition is a relativistic one.

The observer, that is the clinician or researcher, can choose to describe or understand pain phenomena in any of several ways. However, I must caution you that I am *not* referring to what has been called the "multiple-aspects" theory. The essential concept of this idea is diagrammed in Figure 16-3. On the left side, for the sake of convenience, five categories of the many kinds of phenomena listed in Figure 16-1 are given and abstracted into our relativistic definition. These five categories represent different "levels" of pain responses, employ different methods of observations and use different vocabularies referring to different concepts.

It is, therefore, not correct to say that these approaches are merely used to investigate different aspects of the same phenomenon, "pain," because this implies that the pain, as shown on the right side of the diagram, is a single real entity. Pain is not a single entity that we simply describe in different ways. Rather, pain is an abstract term referring to

MULTIPLE − ASPECTS THEORY

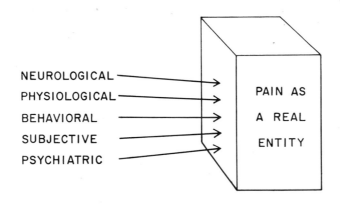

NEUROLOGICAL
PHYSIOLOGICAL
BEHAVIORAL
SUBJECTIVE
PSYCHIATRIC

PAIN AS
A REAL
ENTITY

(DIFFERENT WAYS OF DESCRIBING THE SAME THING)

Figure 16-3

many different real things: different experiences, different stimuli and different responses—all real, but all different.

In Figure 16-4, I have attempted to diagram what seems to me to be the real state of affairs regarding the concept of pain. This I call "linguistic parallelism," expanding on the phrase and concept first proposed by Dr. David T. Graham (1). According to this view, the different approaches to pain (again arbitrarily sorted into five categories for the sake of convenience) are recognized as dealing with somewhat different phenomena. Not only are the methods, concepts and vocabularies different, but some of

LINGUISTIC PARALLELISM (GRAHAM)

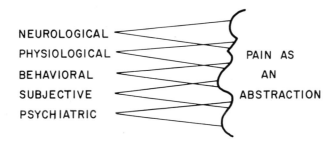

NEUROLOGICAL
PHYSIOLOGICAL
BEHAVIORAL
SUBJECTIVE
PSYCHIATRIC

PAIN AS
AN
ABSTRACTION

DIFFERENT CONCEPTS DESCRIBING SOME DIFFERENT THINGS IN DIFFERENT WAYS)

Figure 16-4

the data are also. The neurophysiological activities attended to by the neurologist are quite different from the responses to catecholamine and steroids observed by the internist, for example. The verbal descriptions or ratings and overt bodily responses that the psychologist measures are likewise a different order of phenomena from the affective or interpersonal responses to which the psychiatrist might address himself. Each of these is in a different class from what the patient himself experiences subjectively.

None of these events has any inherent relationship to any other. It is we who have arbitrarily imposed on all of them the common concept, "pain." If we can remember that there is no single real thing that is pain, but rather that "pain" is an abstract, unifying concept that we ourselves have arbitrarily imposed on a great many different kinds of things, then perhaps we can free ourselves to think and deal more effectively with problems when they arise. There need not be any arguments about which is the "right" approach, because all these parallel approaches are "right." That is, each describes some different things in different ways, and each approach is internally consistent and follows the rules of its own game of investigation.*

To put it another way, it is not any more legitimate or scientific to look at evoked responses from thalamic intralaminar nuclei than it is to listen to a patient's verbal productions. Both are observable and objective data which can be measured, scored, scaled, categorized or in other ways treated in reliable and reproducible ways. We follow one approach rather than another as a matter of personal preference, not because one is more "right" than the other. It is possible to be so invested in looking at only one set of events, however, that the observer misses useful information that comes from looking at others. For example, faced with a patient with persistent phantom limb pain, the neurosurgeon may begin a series of procedures, starting with excision of peripheral neuromas, moving on to a tractotomy and ending with a lobotomy, and never look at the possible affective or interpersonal reasons why the patient needs to have that pain. The psychiatrist would be similarly inflexible if he examined intrapsychic conflicts or interpersonal manipulations and ignored the possibility of stump neuromas. All the approaches provide different information, and

---

* An analogy may be made to the way physicists describe the different phenomena of light. Reflection and the photoelectric effect, for example, require formulas describing the actions of the light particles, photons, whereas such effects as polarization and diffraction require formulas describing wave motion. Still other effects must be described in probabilistic terms. Neither the wave motion theory nor the mechanical theory nor the probabilistic theory can alone describe all the effects of light. Physicists no longer seem to worry about what light *is;* they simply choose the descriptive framework appropriate to the task at hand.

"PSYCHIATRIC" APPROACH TO PAIN REDUCTION

PROBLEM	PRINCIPLE	METHODS
MINIMIZING "NORMAL" PAIN	ANXIETY REDUCTION	ELICITING CONCERNS ENCOURAGING CATHARSIS, EXPLAINING, REASSURING, APPROPRIATE
TREATING "NON-UNDERSTOOD" PAIN.	RELIEVING DEPRESSION	MEDICATIONS, OUTPLAYING "GAME."

Figure 16-5

the approach that is most useful in understanding any particular patient in pain will depend on that patient, not on the scientific disciplines or clinical specialties themselves.

Thus far we have considered three different "strategies," or ways of thinking about pain. The first two assume erroneously that pain is a real thing which either (a) is best understood by a single approach, usually the one we are trained in and by which we make our living, or (b) can be described by different approaches to the same phenomenon. The third strategy, which I am proposing here, is that (c) "pain" is an abstract concept that we use to describe many different phenomena, and we use different languages in doing this.

Now let us consider some of the specific "tactics" available to us if we adopt the last strategy. In Figure 16-5 are outlined what might be called a set of "psychiatric" tactics for reducing or alleviating pain. I put the word "psychiatric" in quotation marks because, as you will see, although the set of tactics derive from traditional psychiatric investigations, the methods themselves are quite varied.

Let us consider first the problem of minimizing "normal" pain, that is pain which is well understood neurologically or which makes sense given the stimuli in the situation. I am thinking of dental drilling or postoperative discomfort or childbirth or serious burns, for example. Preventive measures can greatly minimize the pain responses, and in instances where the patient is already suffering, therapeutic measures can do much to attenuate them. The principle involved is that of reducing anxiety. A great number of studies that are summarized in my book on pain (2) reveal that responses to pain are very similar to those to anxiety, whether these are described in behavioral or subjective or physiological terms. Therefore, any method that reduces anxiety will reduce pain. If anxiety is due to lack of knowledge of the procedure or extent of body harm and implications for future functioning, then psychotherapeutic-like encouragement to express these concerns can be most beneficial when it is followed by appropriate explanations. Similarly, tranquilizers and muscle relaxants, since they interfere with some of the anxiety responses, will likewise diminish pain responses. We are not speaking here of analgesics per se, although it may be that analgesics also work because they decrease anxiety.

The next problem is the difficult one of treating patients who complain of pain that cannot be understood in neurological terms. Such patients may acquire thick hospital charts over the years, as they have one operation after another and make the rounds from doctor to doctor. It is tempting to label them "hysterics" or "crocks," but such labels do not help them nor add to our understanding. Naming, as we know, is not explaining. Now it turns out that psychiatric studies of such patients have found them to be depressed. The depression may result from loss, as in inadequate grief reactions, or it may result from intropunitive reactions, as happens when anger is not appropriately directed outwardly. In chronic conditions such patients become "pain-prone." You must understand that these people are not faking or malingering; they have real pain by any measure we can devise, and their suffering is manifest. But neurological models do not adequately describe them, at least not yet as well as psychiatric ones do. The tactics of treating such patients are those that will relieve depression. This may consist of psychotherapy, which encourages a complete response of mourning or which enables the patient to learn that it is safe and appropriate to express anger directly. Or, if the patient is manipulating or controlling his family with his symptom, family therapy may be necessary to change the system. Or, if therapy is not appropriate for the particular patient, then antidepressant medications, or mood elevators, can be very successful. In fact, for these people with persistent or recurrent pain with no apparent organic basis, analgesics may only worsen their symptoms, whereas antidepressants do much to alleviate them.

Let us consider now the many tactics available for treating patients with chronic pain. These are listed in Figure 16-6 in association with the five approaches we used before, but this is an arbitrary arrangement, there is considerable overlap, and the use of the tactics is really quite independent of origin of the pain.

About surgery and analgesia you know a great deal; these are based on the assumption that pain results from peripheral events that relay impulses cephalad, and if you block the signals you eliminate the pain. While this is true, it is not the only way of thinking about pain, and so other tactics have been evolved to deal with the instances in which these two methods are not appropriate. For example, the "gate-control" model of pain has predicted and confirmed that increasing the input of the

VARIETIES OF TACTICS FOR TREATING CHRONIC PAIN

NEUROLOGICAL
- SURGERY
- ANALGESIA
- INCREASED SENSORY INPUT

PHYSIOLOGICAL
- TRANQUILIZERS
- MUSCLE RELAXANTS
- ANTI-DEPRESSANTS

BEHAVIORAL
- DESENSITIZATION
- AVERSIVE CONDITIONING
- COGNITIVE DISSONANCE

SUBJECTIVE
- HYPNOSIS
- RELIGION
- EXISTENTIALISM

PSYCHIATRIC
- DYNAMIC (DEPRESSION: LOSS; INTROPUNITIVE "PAIN-PRONE")
- OPERANT (NEGATIVE PRACTICE, "PARADOXICAL INTENTIONS")
- FAMILY ("GAMES")

COMMON CONCEPTS:

INPUT: REDUCING "PAIN-LIKE" STIMULI
OUTPUT: ENHANCING INCOMPATIBLE RESPONSES
PRINCIPLE: BREAKING ASSOCIATIVE LINKS

Figure 16-6

classical sensory modalities reduces the transmission along pain fibers. This is the basis for the old "counterirritant" method. In our hospital, Dr. Carl Fellner is setting up a pain laboratory in which patients engage in a variety of motor tasks, with lights flashing and bells ringing, for a half hour or so twice a day. He reports that his preliminary results look rather encouraging, in that complaints of pain appear to diminish over a period of a few weeks.

Tranquilizers, muscle relaxants and antidepressants can be thought of as reducing or interfering with the physiological pain responses, the autonomic and adrenal ones particularly.

Desensitization is a technique of behavior therapy in which the patient learns to substitute relaxation responses to cues that ordinarily would elicit pain responses. This technique has been used successfully in many cases of training for natural childbirth and can be extended to any other situation as well. Aversive conditioning is another behavior therapy technique that can be used to eliminate pain responses; it consists of presenting a strong shock or other noxious stimulus whenever pain behavior appears. Paradoxical as it may seem, it can be used to extinguish the pain responses to the original pain stimuli. Cognitive dissonance techniques

rely on the fact that people must square their beliefs and their behavior;
the patient whose responses are consistently different from pain behavior,
whether relaxation or one of a variety of tasks, must eventually give up
thinking of himself as having pain. Thus, fully programmed activities
can be quite effective.

We can choose to deal directly with the patient's experience rather
than his pain responses. The effectiveness of hypnotic techniques has
long been known and need not be elaborated here. Similarly with patients who have strong religious convictions; it is not for nothing that religion has been called the "opiate of the masses," and the clinician today
should not forget this tactic for separating pain and suffering. Existential
therapists also offer a different approach which tends to "flip" patients.
Instead of asking "Why?" about the pain, the existential therapists ask
"Why not?" The patient who struggles with this issue will either give up
his pain or accept it.

We have already mentioned the therapeutic possibilities of exploring
with the patient the psychodynamics of his depression, whether due to a
real or feared loss or due to anger turned inwards. The operant method,
which might be better categorized as a behavioral technique, consists of
providing the patient control over his pain. He tallies it, makes graphs,
keeps elaborate diaries of the stimuli and events associated with the pain,
and practices deliberately inducing or increasing it. This is a surprisingly
effective method and works quite rapidly. The alteration of pathological
family systems was also mentioned previously. It is referred to as "games,"
not because these are deliberate ways of having fun, but because there
are implicit rules governing role-playing in families, and usually all family members have an unconscious stake in the symptoms of the member
officially designated as the "patient."

If we look at all these tactics for treating chronic pain we can see that
despite their differing vocabularies which describe somewhat different
phenomena, there are certain concepts they have in common. On the input side they serve to reduce pain stimuli or those which, like anxiety
or depression, are sufficiently similar that they potentiate pain stimuli.
On the output side the tactics serve to diminish or extinguish pain behavior directly or indirectly by enhancing behavior that is incompatible
with pain responses.

Considering these effects on input and output, they in turn seem to
share a common principle. Using the vocabulary of conditioning, the principle seems to be one of breaking the associative links between the old
signals and the responses they elicit, which were classed as pain responses.
 Thus *any* technique that dissociates the stimuli and responses, whether

physical, chemical, behavioral or subjective, or whatever, can serve to alleviate pain. We need not be bound by traditions, but are limited only by our imaginations.

In summary, we have examined several strategies or ways of thinking about pain. The one proposed here, called "linguistic parallelism," permits us to feel free and legitimate about looking at different phenomena and the great variety of tactics available for treating them. It turns out that these tactics have certain elements in common: reducing pain-like stimuli, enhancing behavior incompatible with pain responses and, in general, dissociating the established links between inputs and outputs, whatever the vocabulary used.

REFERENCES

1. GRAHAM, D. T.: Health, disease, and the mind-body problem: Linguistic parallelism. *Psychosom Med,* 29:52, 1967.
2. STERNBACH, R. A.: *Pain: A Psychophysiological Analysis.* New York, Academic 1968.

Chapter 17

SOME MEDICOLEGAL ASPECTS OF PAIN, SUFFERING AND MENTAL ANGUISH IN AMERICAN LAW AND CULTURE

Hubert W. Smith

LECTURERS in this symposium have probed deeply into many aspects of pain, suffering and mental anguish. The collective research and impressive clinical data indicate that we are, indeed, on the threshold of new knowledge. Probing ever deeper into the physiology of temporary and permanent forms of this fearsome triad, and into the widely divergent reaction patterns of human beings that are determined psychologically, we must look for all means of alleviating pain, suffering and mental anguish.[1]

In theology, philosophy, medicine, biology and literature, pain, suffering and mental anguish are recurrent themes equated not only with torture and tragedy, but also with faith, hope, charity, character formation, self-effacement and salvation. The causation and cure of pain are but incompletely known to the scientific investigator, and myth, mystery and folk-lore invest the layman's thinking. Well-intentioned lawyers, judges and juries, lacking information, sometimes threaten the evolution of law and its search for justice under the adversary system in cases in which pain is of primary importance.

The views expressed in this paper are in propositional form and suggest the value of interdisciplinary cooperation in an area that involves so much that is *subjective* and so little that can be *qualified* or *quantified* by objective measurement.

---

[1] We should like to see the speculative, subjective phase of personal injury controversies more thoroughly illuminated by knowledgeable specialists in neurology, neurosurgery, psychiatry and psychology, either by joint agreement of opposing counsel for a medicolegal audit, upon which approximate truth could be reached as a basis for pretrial compromise settlement (over 90 percent of cases when handled by experienced lawyers), or as admissible evidence should trial be required. It is believed that the trial judge has inherent jurisdiction to appoint impartial experts, but a better plan is to call upon an independent scientific agency, such as the New York Academy of Medicine in New York, to select the specialists by a "blind" rotation method. An example of impartial medical testimony is given in a Report by a Special Committee of The Association of the Bar of the City of New York, on the Medical Expert Testimony Project. No expert witness should be sponsored as the court's, because this is an indication of infallibility, which is unfair to other experts.

The law seeks to protect interests of personality from culpable injury by others, including both intentional and negligent wrongs as defined by the common law (or judge-made law of torts), as modified or extended by statutes (state or federal). The countenance of any branch of the law may be changed quickly by legislation. The fields of private law and subjects of state concern belong to state legislatures; those of national concern are dealt with by congressional legislation. The Federal Constitution forbids the infliction of cruel and inhuman punishments; and, many believe that this will eventually cause the United States Supreme Court to outlaw the death penalty.[2]

Judges of appellate courts, whose opinions are preserved, printed, studied and cited as precedents, establish legal principles more extensively, perhaps, than those of any other courts, seeking to fit evolving rights and duties to dictates of social needs and conscience. Suffice it to say that the law first protected man and his property against culpable physical injury, as from trespass or assault and battery, requiring the wrongdoer to compensate his victim for material losses inflicted. It is only in recent times that we have had a burgeoning of legal protection accorded to psychic interests of personality. The first treatise in English on torts was published in 1859. Today, court decisions are legion; and, law review articles, comments and notes are multitudinous (see Index to Legal Periodicals). There are various publications having to do with particular torts such as defamation, fraud, personal injuries, products liability and aviation and maritime accidents. There are special fields such as workmen's compensation statutes which do not require proof of fault, but only that the workman received a personal injury as the result of an accident sustained in the course and scope of employment. Other torts relate to the expanding field of family law.

---

[2] The eighth amendment to the Federal Constitution prohibits the infliction of cruel and inhuman punishments, but this applies only to federal courts. Death penalties imposed by state courts might well have to be attacked as violations of the fourteenth amendment (due process clause) (*In re Kimmler*, 136 U.S. 436, 10 S. Ct. 930, 34 L. Ed. 519, is an old case in which the Federal Supreme Court held death by electrocution not to be a cruel punishment). The Supreme Court might well now hold that the due process clause reenacts the Bill of Rights, including the eighth amendment, and rule differently when the assigned error is supported by strong psychological evidence that shows capital punishment is cruel. We raised this proposition in the second amended motion for new trial in *State of Texas vs. Jack Ruby*, but the conviction was reversed, on other grounds, by the Texas Court of Criminal Appeals, and Ruby died of cancer before a new trial. We assume that, undoubtedly this proposition will be raised in appeal of *State of California vs. Sirhan*, and sooner or later will be passed upon by the United States Supreme Court. In the Jack Ruby Case we offered expert testimony that the anxiety of anticipated execution is more punishing and painful than infliction of physical pain, which the high court earlier held to be unconstitutional (*Weems vs. United States*, 217 U.S. 349, 30 S. Ct. 544, 54 L. Ed. 793, 19 Ann. Cas. 705).

In the past, awards of damages to compensate wrongfully inflicted pain, suffering and mental anguish were limited. Juries were ultraconservative, and both trial and appellate judges were not averse to holding a verdict excessive and awarding a new trial for passion and prejudice unless the plaintiff reduced or waived the allegedly excessive part of his recovery under the doctrine of *remittitur*. Today, pain, dramatically presented to a jury, may be the basis for a very large award, shocking to no one but the defendant. This phenomenon, now in need of close scrutiny and intelligent regulation, results from a new humanistic philosophy and an explosive extension of protection given to expanding interests of personality. Furthermore, legal protection against wrongful infliction of pain has not only risen vertically, but has spread laterally to embrace pain, suffering and mental anguish in infinite ramifications. This protection covers every variety of pain known to neurologists, neurosurgeons and psychiatrists. It embraces referred pain, phantom limb pain and involvement of body image, and more recently complaints of a psychological nature. Casualty insurance companies often do not complain concerning high damages in catastrophic injury cases, but rather object to the frequency of $10,000 awards for chronic low-back pain and persistent complaints following uncomplicated soft tissue injuries of the neck. The battles of trial technique are promoted by the lack of any definite standards by which a jury can measure the compensation to be awarded. As McCormick said, "Translating pain and anguish into dollars can, at best, be only an arbitrary allowance, and not a process of measurement, and consequently the judge can, in his instructions, give the jury no standard; he can only tell the jurymen to allow such amount as in their discretion they may consider reasonable."

There is a pressing need for studies dealing with the relationships of physical and psychological trauma to the various organ systems of the body, as well as to the total personality. Scientific criteria of proof are needed with respect to such matters as primary causation of injury or disability by trauma, aggravation of preexisting conditions and precipitation of latent disease. This summary cannot attempt to offer such proof. Rather, it is merely intended to convey certain scientific insights that are believed to be medically well founded but which may yet be unfamiliar to the legal scholar or trial lawyer. There are possibly as many as 100,000 articles appearing annually in medical and scientific journals throughout the world. There is at present no adequate means for screening and evaluating this torrential flow to determine its authenticity and social and legal relevancy. Scientific progress is accelerating, and the findings of yesterday are, in some cases, obsolete today. Medical literature produced only a few years ago is often obsolete. The literature is thus a grab bag of innumerable articles of variable quality and authority, tempting to the alert advocate who seeks to support a special theory. One solution is to marshal, in law-science institutions, the most eminent specialists and investigators available and to nurture philosophies and procedures that may bring the rule of science into the administration of justice. For example, such an organization as The Law-Science Academy might, in cooperation with specialists from medical centers, develop selected and current bibliographies that could be attached to written interrogatories or depositions.

In these efforts to insure proof, we must not lose sight of the fact that proof-making does not occur in a vacuum. Human beings must weigh the evidence, and there are several components of unequal probative value that play upon the minds of the triers of fact. Evidence has both persuasive and probative value, and, unfortunately, these may not lead the inquiring mind in the same direction. These reflections force the conclusion that in the field of proof, corroboration by diverse types of evidence may be exceedingly important.

The perpetuation of our adversary system may well depend upon its ability to bring scientific justice to the contending parties. This, in turn, may depend not only on continuing development of "the proofs of science," but upon the training of true law-science advocates, competent to handle scientific evidence in evaluating cases for settlement or in trying disputed issues in court. It is our belief that the adversary system of trial can and will evolve to meet this standard of justice. It is in this spirit that we offer a few observations in fields in which subjective factors make objective proofs virtually unattainable.

One of the most speculative factors upon which triers of fact must place a monetary value is pain and suffering. There are receptors for pain in the skin, muscles, joints and other tissues. In addition, when other types of receptors are overstimulated, the subject may also feel pain. Experiments to quantitate pain have aroused considerable interest, but these tests are not truly objective because the investigator must rely on the veracity of the subject, and the theory that all subjects have the same threshold to pain is not tenable at this time.

It might be assumed that lawyers have been guilty of their often-suspected indulgence in prolixity, redundancy and meaningless similes in using the three terms "pain, suffering and mental anguish." Each of these conditions involves a disagreeable invasion of emotional and intellectual tranquillity. Yet it would seem that each term may have a broad scope of distinctive meaning not necessarily covered by the other two.

Thus, the perception of "pain" involves lower levels. "Suffering" embraces the various modalities of psychological and clinical reaction and depends upon personality structure, life-conditioning, philosophy and perhaps individual differences in secondary neural mechanisms. Suffering may be protean in character, embracing an amazing range of psychologically disagreeable sensations and symptoms, such as anxiety, hallucinations, delusions, insomnia, catastrophic dreams, fears, worry, hate, guilt and disagreeable displacements or distortions of usual emotions, sensations or bodily reactions. "The various forms of mental suffering are as numberless as the capacities of the human soul for torturing itself."[3] Suffering may persist after pain has gone. Many traumatic neurosis cases follow a psychic stimulus wrongfully applied rather than from physical injury. Indeed, it is rather well agreed that it is the psychological effect of the accident rather than physical injury which triggers traumatic neurosis. With respect to "mental anguish," we are dealing less with pain and subsequent suffering than with psychological conscious discomfort involving a sense of social alienation, as may occur from disfiguring or deforming injuries that might follow catastrophic burns. The law now extends its rights of compensatory redress, by way of damages, to each variety of conscious pain, suffering and mental anguish. The law has also now brought into the realm of compensable injury the consequences of unconscious sensory and motor impulses that result in so-called "psychosomatic" injuries, diseases or symptoms.

While the initial perception of pain might seem to be fairly uniform, elements of interpretation and association are involved, so that the reaction of any individual to pain and its meaning for him are highly subjective, depending upon his personality structure and prior conditioning. Thus, the meaning and interpretation of pain and the way in which it is perceived is an individual experience, highly subjective and virtually indefinable. The problem posed is similar to that of asking a person to describe the color "red." The pain and suffering felt by a particular individual in response to a uniform stimulus may vary greatly from that felt by others. Some persons are nonresponsive to pain, some are average reactors and some are hypersensitive.

---

[3] Hickenbottom vs. Delaware, L. & W. R. Co., 122 N. Y. 91, 25 N. E. 279 (1890). A claim for bodily pain is held to make proof of mental suffering automatically admissible. Courts have held compensable as mental suffering: the claimant's fright and terror at the time of his injury; reasonable apprehension concerning future effects upon his or her health (fear of cancer following burns, set up by warnings of treating dermatologist); apprehension of a pregnant woman that her unborn child has been injured; anxiety over inability to earn a living; fear of death or insanity as a result of injury; traumatic neuroses, sadness, humiliation, embarrassment and mental anguish resulting from scars, mutilation or disfiguring injuries.

Conditioning will have a bearing upon an individual's tolerance of pain or his tendency to feel it acutely and complain about it. It has been reported that certain racial types seem to complain more of pain than others. Further complicating this task is the fact that physical and psychological factors may alter the pain response even in a given person at different times. Pain may be felt more acutely by one who is fatigued, nervous or distressed; or, when factors cause the subject to focus his attention upon the painful experience. On the other hand, the perception of pain may be greatly reduced when attention is distracted.

Pain can be a protective function. It is often a danger signal. Serious injuries may befall a person who has lost his receptivity to pain. An individual with leprosy may burn his hand without realizing that injury is being done until he smells the burning flesh. In like manner, a normal individual who sustains serious third degree burns may suffer little pain, because the nerve endings are destroyed.

In our Judeo-Christian heritage it has sometimes been argued that pain should be regarded as punishment. The concept of hell involves infliction of pain. Civilized nations may permit capital punishment, yet forbid the infliction of pain upon the criminal. Masochists are individuals who derive pleasure from having pain inflicted upon themselves. Still other individuals gain great psychological satisfaction from their Spartan-like ability to withstand pain or privation. Some philosophers have argued that life would lose its savor if it were without pain, and that pain serves to increase the appreciation of pleasures, by contrast, and to enrich and deepen the human personality. But while pain may have an ennobling influence and refine the character of the sufferer, very few individuals would voluntarily choose this mode of personality development.

Pain may often be accompanied by collateral reactions such as anxiety. Many psychoanalysts agree that the mental anguish that the neurotic experiences as the result of his anxieties are more punishing than any type of physical pain. This leads to the question of whether pain is always transient, or may sometimes be permanent. It would seem that once the stimulus that initiates pain is removed, the response will cease. Most neurologists agree that there are very few traumatic injuries that produce permanent pain. In most instances, then, pain is temporary. To support a claim of long-continuing or permanent pain, one needs to find some explanation, such as chronic irritation, or traumatic arthritis in a weight-bearing joint where continued pressure traumatizes the painful member. The limited duration of most traumatic pain has never been appreciated properly, nor capitalized upon, by defense counsel. Physicians often search for "objective" signs of pain. Muscle spasm, dilation of the pupils and elevation of temperature may give objective evidence of reflex response to painful stimuli.

The conduct of a person may have corroborating value. Some individuals complain about a terrific headache, and yet do so with a smiling face. Physicians refer to these as "happy headaches" and do not rate the pain as severe. Other patients may give every evidence by their conduct that they are suffering real and punishing pain calling for administration of analgesics or narcotics. If the pain is sufficiently severe, plaintiff's counsel may be able to argue that his client cannot get relief without narcotics, and that if he takes such drugs, he stands in danger of addiction.

In certain courts it has been accepted that the greater the wound, the greater the resultant pain. The Supreme Court of Texas has held this to be so well-known that it requires no supporting evidence. This is an untenable assumption. The degree of pain depends upon a number of factors. Some areas of the body have many more pain receptors in a given area than do other parts and are therefore more pain-sensitive. A small lesion may produce great pain, while a much larger wound may produce relatively little pain.

Most lawyers have known of cases in which individuals sustained exsanguinating injuries that led rapidly to shock and death. In these cases, the argument is often made in support of damages for conscious pain and suffering that the individual's pain was greatly intensified and that such a person might well have felt great anguish in reviewing his entire life in the few minutes before he expired. Actually, we know that when an injury is sufficient to create a state of shock, the sensorium is dulled. The individual becomes oblivious to pain and may be almost immune to conscious suffering. This, again, is a fact that is often not known to defense counsel.

Let us turn now to another subject of special importance in determining individual response to physical or psychological trauma. We refer here to the pretraumatic personality or character of the individual plaintiff. The pretraumatic personality structure of a victim has a material bearing upon his reactions to injury and disability, as well as to the prospects of his successful rehabilitation. A review of the literature indicates that the personality of the victim is indeed an important determinant of the effects of the trauma. From this one might infer that it is possible to categorize types of personality and that each of these types will react predictably to a specific traumatic episode. Unfortunately, reliable patterns of predictability have not yet emerged. There are certain features that seem to comprise the posttraumatic syndrome or postconcussion syndrome. These features are exhibited when the individual reacts adversely to injury or disability, regardless of personality type in the usual sense of the word. The various types of personality classifications are based largely upon a surface description of the individual's characteristic traits; for example, the classification of two types of personality: the extrovert and the introvert. Another type of classification is a labeling of various personality types to compare with psychiatric disorders. Thus, there are schizoid, paranoid, compulsive and cyclothymic personalities. All of these classifications are essentially descriptive, and one searches in vain for a specific type of traumatic response that the individual characterized as one of these personality patterns may be expected to develop.

Another way of regarding personality types seems to be more useful and to hold greater promise in evaluating the problems of causation and prognosis. This is the so-called "dynamic approach," which has come to the fore in recent years as the basic analytical rationale of modern psychiatry. The term "dynamic" refers to the energies involved in the operation or functioning of the personality. The interplay of these energies or forces results in the personality of the individual.

Involved in the development of the personality is the reconciliation of the demands and pressures of the outside world with the individual's inner drives and cravings. As a part of the educational process, the infant learns to give as well as to take. As the child gets older, the basic pattern of outside requirements becomes known to him and he selects various ways of fitting the pattern. He finally develops a self-regulating device by which he guides his own behavior. This involves a series of private meanings, codes and formulations taken from the patterns of persons who have at earlier times influenced his life. His special recombinations make him unique.

In the development of the personality of a particular individual, the need to be cared for, which we all feel as small children, may fail to come into a healthy balance with the opposing need to achieve independence and self-assertiveness. An individual with such a personality may devise ways of acquiring extra protection that have gone unnoticed by others. An example of this is the individual who continues at school not so much for the purpose of obtaining an education as to prolong the time he is dependent upon his family. Posttraumatically, this kind of person may exhibit clinging helplessness, demand more and more care and continue to complain of weakness and tiredness. He is secure in the care he is receiving and seeks to prolong it.

Another personality type may be one who regards a strong healthy body as his most important asset. Injury, although only temporary, may result in the traumatic expression of a limp or a stooped posture, emphasizing the change that has come over his body. To the objective medi-

cal examiner he may have a vigorous young physique, but he stays at
home with complaints of pain that serve to call attention to the fact that
he can no longer depend upon the body that he had felt to be his chief
security.

Anxiety is a very powerful force. It has the capacity to make an individual sick, to prolong disability and even to kill on occasion. Furthermore, it is a frame of mind that is present to some degree in all injuries.
Each injury or disability has its particular meaning for the injured person. Just as factors in the environment may focus attention upon the
painful lesion and increase suffering, or distract attention from it and
lessen the anguish. so internal factors may serve to intensify or diminish
pain.

Physiological changes induced by great and sudden fright, mobilizing
the organism for "fight-flight" reactions, tend to be short-lived. Once the
immediate threat or the frightening stimulus is removed, the organism
tends to go back to a resting phase. Injury ascribed to fright, on a physiological basis, must occur within a very short time of the cessation of the
frightening stimulus in order for there to be causal relationship. Psychological reactions evolve more slowly, may be more complex and may constitute true effects, though delayed at the time of their onset. It is our
belief that anxiety is the central symptom in any neurosis.

It would seem clear that multiple factors enter any reaction to pain,
injury or disability. These might be listed as follows: (a) event itself—
that is to say, the nature of the stimulus applied; (b) nature and circumstances of the injury or disability; (c) factor of anxiety; (d) noncon-
scious elements; (e) factor of compensation; and (f) personality of the
individual.

Nature of the Stimulus Applied

It is well known that the nature of physical or psychological trauma
may have a direct bearing upon the immediate and remote consequences. There are various consequences that may be precipitated by
fright. The psychological import of the stimulus (rather than physical
injury) may be the cause of neuroses following trauma. Most, if not
all, individuals who manifest a posttraumatic neurosis have catastrophic dreams in which they relive the frightening experience. The
degree of a physical injury may also be determined by the nature of
the physical stimulus. Thus, in a scientific study of traumatology it is
necessary to investigate fully the nature and import of the traumatic
stimulus and the period during which it was applied. It is assumed at
this time that the "functional" psychoses (such as schizophrenia and
manic-depressive psychosis) are not due to organic injury of the ner-

vous system. Nevertheless, cases have been cited by reputable investigators where these conditions have been precipitated in a person inclined to a given psychosis, or previously hospitalized with it, and it has been generally believed that it is the psychological import of the incident that has a greater influence than any physical lesion. An example is the case of a young woman with an unwanted pregnancy who was involved in an automobile accident. Although not seriously injured, she developed a psychosis attributed by the attending psychiatrist to her guilt feelings about her former death wishes toward the child.

Nature of the Injury

In like manner, injury or disability may have a private meaning for the particular subject. This may be the determining factor as to what the final effect will be. The event itself may not be severe, but the reaction may be extreme. For example, an automobile accident occurred in which the subject's head was struck, but he was not rendered unconscious and showed no evidence of physical injury. Nevertheless, the individual exhibited concern for years about even the slightest symptoms referable to a state of unconsciousness and complained of dizziness, absentmindedness and near blackouts. These symptoms became more understandable when it was learned that in an automobile accident the victim's father had suffered an injury following which he had developed severe convulsive seizures which occurred intermittently for the rest of his life. The seizures caused the father to lose his position and to be unable to get another, so that his ability to support his family was completely destroyed. The meaning of the accident to our subject then was the important thing in determining his reactions to it, and the actual severity of the injury had less to do with the patient's reaction than the private meanings.

The part of the body involved may also be of some significance. It is well known that various parts of the body have different values for most people, and in a definite order, with the genitals and the head at the top of the list. Then come the upper extremities, the legs, back and other parts of the body. Nor should one overlook the fact that jurors share with the victims of injury and disability the same concern about the various parts of the body.

Factor of Anxiety

Anxiety is a very potent force that may increase in intensity after the immediate emergency is over. Anxiety seems to be an inevitable consequence of injury and disability. It is repressed rapidly by various psychological devices at the subject's disposal. It serves, for the most part unconsciously, as the foundation for the reaction to the injury or disability. The symptoms may be sensations. Most commonly, pain is the complaint. This may be headache, in the case of head and neck injuries, or pain referable to the particular organ system involved. Thus, one may have prolonged pain referred to fractures that have long since healed. Other sensations that may be the source of complaints are dizziness, blurring of vision and internal sensations such as nausea.

Usually, the sensation will be appropriate to the nature and location of the trauma and injury. Disturbances in mobility as well as disturbances in sensation may occur. This is particularly true of the extremities, where an injury may result in marked reduction in the movability of the part. Lack of movement may bear little relationship to the extent of the tissue damaged and may reflect some particular psychological meaning that the part has for its owner. Further, the signs of anxiety usually appear in the absence of anxiety as a complaint. The anxiety may be translated into other symptoms that form a part of the posttraumatic reaction, such as sweaty palms, periods of rapid breathing and rapid heart rate, loss of appetite and uneasiness. All of these, in point of fact, may be manifestations of anxiety and may persist and be complained of by the patient without his acknowledgement of anxiety. In addition to this, anxiety itself may appear only in response to other symptoms caused by the injury or reactions to it—the headache, the backache and the like—driving the individual from one physician to another in an attempt to get some relief or an explanation of his complaints.

Nonconscious Elements

The anxiety generated by a traumatic experience operates nonconsciously. This is a difficult thing for most people to accept, for they like to believe that at all times they are fully aware of their own motives and could, if they wished, consciously reconstruct the full background and causes of their behavior. Investigators of human behavior realize that this is not true. Psychological reactions to injuries and disabilities are often prolonged and keep the context of the injury alive in the thoughts of the victim for months or even years.

Factor of Compensation

Of concern to all is the effect of financial compensation in generating a posttraumatic syndrome, and the effect of continued payments for disability in maintaining a posttraumatic reaction. A study of this subject discloses that compensation has something to do with the production and maintenance of posttraumatic syndromes. Of forty-five articles on posttraumatic neuroses, twenty-eight indicated that compensation contributed to the production of a posttraumatic syndrome and to the maintenance of symptoms; no view on this was expressed in sixteen papers; only one study ended with the conclusion that compensation was not a factor in the majority of cases. Many of the authors pointed out that compensation may represent various types of secondary gain (the control of anxiety being the primary gain) in these reactions, quite aside from money and the security that money represents. That is to say that compensation might represent retribution against a hated employer, or payment finally exacted for long periods of indignities suffered at the hands of a hated foreman, etc.

Personality of the Individual

The importance of private values and meanings that the victim may attach to various stresses or injuries has been mentioned. In addition, the pretraumatic personality or character of the accident victim is one of the most influential factors in determining not only whether he will develop adverse reactions, but the form that these will take if they do ensue.

We have been concerned primarily with reactions sometimes called posttraumatic neurosis, the posttraumatic reaction or the traumatic syndrome. Symptoms that develop from organic injury of the nervous system and those that are psychological in origin are quite different. Evaluation may depend upon the combined expertise of the neurologist, electroencephalographer, psychiatrist, clinical psychologist and general physician, and from knowledge gained from family and associates. This leads us back to the theme suggested in the beginning of this paper: the essence of proof, or disproof, is corroboration, and difficult medicolegal cases may require the cooperation and combined knowledge of several specialists in arriving at a thoroughly documented rational conclusion.

According to English common law, it was a compensable wrong to physically injure one's fellow man by a wrongful act or omission; but, if the victim died, neither his administrator nor his surviving relatives could maintain any action for damages. This anomaly was partially corrected by Lord Campbell's Act, enacted in England in 1846 (the Fatal Accidents Act), preserving only a part of the victim's original cause of action to his dependents as "pecuniary loss." Subsequently, various American states added separate "Survival Statutes," preserving to the victim's administrator elements of damage occurring before death; but, these, too, are imperfect, for some jurisdictions do not permit actions to be brought under both statutes for the same act or omission.

Today, many American states have removed limiting ceilings from their "Wrongful Death Statutes." Still others have broadened the scope of recoverable damages from loss of earnings and services of a minor child, wrongfully killed by defendant, to embrace such items as sums expended in rearing and educating the child, and even damages to the parents for psychic factors, such as loss of the child as an object of love, affection and companionship.

An historic case in extending legal protection to impairment of health and the pleasures of life is *Fair vs. The London and Northwestern Railway Co.*, decided in England in 1869 by Chief Justice Cockburn. Here a twenty-seven-year-old unmarried minister, possessed of excellent health and earning £250 a year, was seriously injured in a train wreck. Evidence showed that the accident culpably caused by the defendant made the plaintiff permanently deaf, injured his spine—causing permanent paralysis of the lower extremities and some impairment of sensation—and converted him into a helpless invalid for the remainder of his life. The Appeals Court held that the jury's award of damages might properly include consequences of shattered health in addition to mere economic losses.[4] This raises the further question of whether a person has a psychic interest in continuation of his own life, so that compensatory damages may be recovered for defendant's culpable behavior resulting in wrongful shortening of plaintiff's life expectancy.

Thus, the pain-pleasure plexus gained legal protection before Freud introduced these considerations in his psychoanalytic models of hypothetical psychodynamics.

The fascinating American case of *Robinson vs. Utility Company*[5] is one of many American cases that have recently upheld loss or impairment of

[4] The jury, in *Fair vs. Ry.*, returned a verdict allowing plaintiff general damages of £5,000 and £250 for medical and other expenses. In denying a motion for a new trial on the ground of excessive damages, the Court said:

"Now the rule is that where a railway company undertakes to carry a passenger and he receives an injury in consequence of their negligence, he is entitled to receive compensation from them, and in assessing that compensation the jury should take into account two things; first, the pecuniary loss he sustains by the accident; secondly, the injury he sustains to his person, or his physical capacity of enjoying life. When they come to the consideration of the pecuniary loss, they have to take into account not only his personal loss but his incapacity to earn a future improved income. . . . Then as to the second ground, undoubtedly health is the greatest of all physical blessings; and to say that when it is utterly shattered, no compensation is to be made for it is really perfectly extravagant."

[5] In this case, a family man who romped with his children and pursued the pleasures of life with vigor was suddenly converted into a paraplegic by an accident found to have been negligently caused. The defendant had used a telephone pole rotten at its base. As the plaintiff lineman climbed to make repairs, the pole snapped, and the fall severed his spinal cord. In upholding a jury award for more than $225,000, the Florida Court scarcely mentioned loss of wages, but dwelt almost exclusively on pain, suffering, mental anguish, deprivation of the pleasure of good health and destruction of the social existence of a victim in the prime of life.

the pleasures of life wrongfully caused by defendant's conduct as a proper element of damages in personal injury actions.

In the past I have contended that the Components of Proof include six factors, in cases tried before a judge or jury, namely:

1. Preconceptions of the Trier of Fact;
2. Psychological components;
3. The factual component;
4. Legal component;
5. Logical component;
6. Scientific component.

Personally, we believe that jury trial by highly trained men of integrity is best calculated to bring out the truth and to secure justice in civil or criminal trials. At the same time, closure of the gap between law and science is impeded by certain indisputable facts:

1. Our Courts hold that any possessor of a doctorate in medicine is competent to testify on any medical subject, extending his knowledge by reading if he has had no personal experience with the problem at hand. This causes many who are motivated by love, sympathy, cupidity, ignorance or greed to make a shambles of science in their testimony.
2. Corroboration is the essence of proof. This includes the opinions of impartial experts in all controversies of any moment.

In the advocate system current ethics permit "fee-splitting," so that the referring lawyer may properly receive one-half of the final fee. This encourages the trial lawyer of moderate ability to associate "big name" advocates who are nationally known for the results they have gained in particular sorts of litigation. We cannot expect advocates to neglect any component of proof—least of all the psychology of persuasion, when human beings rather than computers evaluate evidence, hear arguments and apply legal principles to reach verdicts.[6]

It is interesting that a scientist should say: "The difference is simple, law seeks justice whereas science seeks truth." This represents a remarkable splitting of social goals. Yet it is true that justice is commonly

---

[6] Persons with broad knowledge, and devoid of social bias, recognize that unilateral investigations or administrative proceedings are not as effectual as the adversary system in bringing all relevant evidence to light. Truly great trial lawyers are not dedicated to suppressing truth, nor interested in distorting facts, betraying justice or making the worse appear the better reason. Their facilities for investigating facts are remarkable; even more superb is the sharpness of their dissecting scalpel in cross-examination. Wigmore, master of the Law of Evidence, once said: "Cross-examination is the greatest engine ever invented by man for the discovery of truth."

thought of as a jury's expression of the community conscience. Law students are often reminded: "A Fact is only an opinion that cannot be dislodged by any presently available form of proof." Jurors wish to identify with science and truth, and we are obliged to provide them with components of proof that will lead them to make just decisions.

There are powerful pragmatic reasons, conversely, why we must preserve the interests of personality now recognized by law and society, without permitting these interests to become uncontrollable elements of damages. The legally protected interests of personality, gained through "blood, sweat and tears," cannot be sacrificed for business profits. Scientific guidance and cooperation are necessary in developing criteria and limits for compensation of physical and psychic injuries. Such cooperation will effect quick adjudication, and encourage rehabilitation programs, will catalyze production of scientifically trained trial lawyers, equitable handling of personal injury claims, protection of the casualty insurer's solvency, curtailment of avoidable torts and injuries, and the solution of problems of fault and the uninsured. Accident prevention and consumer protection are other matters that deserve the attention of medicolegal experts.

Contending arguments made by opposing counsel concerning pain in personal injury cases are pertinent to this symposium. The counsel serving the plaintiff dwells upon the fact that the Bible depicts the pain of "hell-fire and brimstone" as the greatest punishment the sinner may undergo in afterlife. He deepens resentment against the defendant by seeking to show that the patient went to the physician with a chief complaint of pain; that the torture suffered has been long-continued and may be permanent; and that pain is evil and destructive and forecloses enjoyment of previous pleasures. The plaintiff himself is urged to see the doctor often, to make diary entries of every minute species of pain he feels or have his family and social contacts testify as to grimaces, groans and changes in personality. The counsel stresses the addictive qualities of many pain-relieving drugs. Described vividly are the patient's saddened life, hospital stay and confinement at home with the anxieties and fears he feels, including the psychic travail. Writers of texts on trial technique in proving pain and suffering stress that each case must be made into a carefully progressing drama, based on hospital or medical procedures and designed to have maximal emotional impact upon the jurors.[7]

[7] Chapman's "Pain and Suffering" (a part of *Courtroom Medicine,* L. Gelfand; and R. D. Magana, Eds. Bender, Albany, 1967) is a treatise on pain by a psychologist, interlarded with plaintiff-oriented trial technique for maximizing jury verdicts. It would appear that medically trained writers (identity unknown) have been used freely to deal with problems falling within the domain of neurological sciences and the medical and surgical specialties. The work contains some useful medical references, but very little identification of legal "case histories" and scarcely any legal documentation.

Defense counsel, conversely, seeks to discredit claims concerning the existence, intensity or permanence of pain. He dwells upon pain-relieving drugs and procedures. He may offer motion pictures of the claimant, showing him performing exertions he has testified are impossible because of pain involved. These reveal that the plaintiff is deriving pleasure from what he does and that he is free of pain; or, it may be pointed out that character is built through pain, suffering and adversity.

Each counsel may use clinical psychologists and psychiatrists to illuminate the claimant's personality structure and verify conflicting contentions as to the existence, nature and degree of his client's pain, suffering and mental anguish.[8]

The law is equally committed to the twin principles designed to achieve justice for society as a whole, and for the individual with respect to compensation of legally protected interests of personality against wrongful, injurious invasion.

It must be remembered that the wrongdoer takes his victim as he finds him, and cannot complain if the particular claimant was more vulnerable to the injurious stimulant—whether because of his age, poor health, prior disease, accident, infirmity, defective inheritance or environment. By the same token, a defendant cannot be made to answer in damages for a preexisting injury, disease, defect or disability the claimant already had. The plaintiff must prove that defendant's conduct primarily caused, precipitated or aggravated the condition for which he seeks compensation.

Extremely broad legal protection of interests of personality is now generally accepted. Many practicing advocates are masters of persuasive arts as well as of probative evidence. This "increased compassion," resulting in ever-mounting verdicts, raises premium costs of automobile and other casualty insurance to impractical levels. Since pain, suffering and mental anguish are subjective, they tend to become uncontrollable factors under present mechanisms of trial and social conscience. They may even threaten the continuation of jury trial in civil cases. It is thus urgent that moderating methods be designed to achieve equity based upon the best that scientific evidence can offer.

A very serious question is presented as to how the conscientious individual physician can play a role in effectively promoting this concept of justice. The naiveté of some reformers was revealed in the "Minnesota plan," based on the assumption that every doctor knows all of the an-

---

[8] We have no fault to find with this, provided the experts are truly competent and unbiased, are used as auxiliary witnesses only and are subjected to penetrating cross-examination by Law-Science advocates thoroughly familiar with the contributions and limitations of those fields and current authoritative literature.

swers to vexatious medical problems if he only tells the truth. The Minnesota plan called for a system of auditing trials, or perusing the statement of facts, to determine whether physicians had spoken truly or falsely. Departure from accepted standards might invite censure or even loss of license. The truth of the matter is that ignorance is a greater foe of justice than fraud. It is no reflection upon the physician that medical information far exceeds individual capacity. Medicine is now divided into more than thirty specialties, each of which requires years of postgraduate training. Specialists, for the most part, must limit themselves to the literature of their fields in order to be aware of recent developments. It would be unrealistic to expect that members of the medical profession would reach complete agreement in solving any medical problem. Much in the field of medical science necessarily involves opinion and even hypothesis. Thus, the difference of opinion among specialists who are essentially in agreement may be marshalled into conflicting medical briefs by eager advocates. Parts of the truth may be mistaken for the whole. Prejudice can result when a judge throws a mantle of omniscience over a court-appointed expert. Though we personally favor the use of such medical experts, they should be brought into court without official sponsorship.

What, then, is needed to fully develop "the proofs of science and the science of proof" that will profitably utilize the learning and experience of medical men and associated scientists, and which will lead to more scientific fact-finding processes? We suggest the following:

1. Trial judges should be slow, on *voir dire* examination, to qualify general practitioners as opinion experts on subjects that are within the realm of medical specialties.
2. The attending physician, even though he be a general practitioner, should always be allowed to testify on the basis of personal knowledge as to what he did, saw and heard, and to give his opinion based upon personal attendance and treatment.
3. Adequate instruction in the field of forensic medicine, designed to meet the needs of all aspiring trial lawyers, should be instituted in law schools. Postgraduate training should be made available to practicing trial counsels. The ideal would be to create a body of law-science advocates, both for plaintiff and defense.
4. There should be an attempt to develop systematically "the proofs of science and the science of proof." While nonprofit organizations such as the Law-Science Academy of America have set up training centers, a great deal of support is needed to enable law students, young lawyers and judges to attend and obtain instruction.

5. Scientific investigators and clinicians should be encouraged to study controversial issues involving relationships of injury to disease and disability. More information must be accumulated to develop criteria of proof that can be made available to physicians who may be called upon to testify upon these repetitive issues.

6. There is a need for some authoritative law-science publication. Leading men in the various medical specialties could serve as associate editors, helping to screen and evaluate the pertinent medical literature and determine its validity and usefulness in social and legal considerations. Such men would cooperate in preparation of original articles designed to evaluate controversial issues and to help create reasonable criteria of proof.

7. The old common-law theory of a "conflict in the evidence" must be reconsidered. The apparent conflict between the opinion of a general practitioner and of a specialist is illusory. The standards of the hospital and medical school must be brought into the courtroom. If a trial judge errs in qualifying a man tendered as an expert, he may later rectify the mistake by cancelling the testimony and dismissing the physician from the stand, as he has continuing surveillance of expert testimony throughout the trial.

8. Insurance companies should recognize their trustee obligation to see that the limited funds available for compensation of injuries are paid as fairly as possible. Unfortunately, while many of the large casualty companies have complained of inflated or unjust verdicts, they have not joined in any militant campaign to counteract this trend. They must be assured that their defense counsels have adequate, continuing instruction in the law-science area. They need, along with the philanthropic foundations of the country, to help finance scholarships for young, promising law students who could be trained in the principles of law-science advocacy.

9. Pretrial discovery of every sort needs to be enhanced, even though trial by jury is not outmoded. The full flowering of the "science of proof" should not be in the courtroom, but at the stage of compromise, negotiation and settlement. This would relieve congestion of the courts and greatly reduce the undesirable hardships that may develop if justice is long delayed. Contending advocates should follow the philosophy and practice of using the finest available experts, of counseling with these experts and of seeking out the lines of corroboration that make fact-finding more secure and certain. Exchange of medical reports and information is necessary to bring about effective compromise negotiation.

10. Contending counsels might mutually agree upon a "medicolegal audit" if they feel they have a good prospect of compromising the liability aspects of a personal injury case, but are in wide disagreement concerning the fact and degree of injury or disability. Under such a procedure both counsels would agree to submit the patient to thorough examination, with the understanding that the medical findings, conclusions and opinions would be reported to both sides. It would further be agreed that the case should be settled upon the basis of these findings, if possible, but that if either party prefers to go to trial, the findings of the medicolegal audit could be offered in evidence without objection, with each party free to offer additional medical testimony. Such a mechanism would help materially to bring an authoritative element into the field of medical evidence.

11. There is an acute need for greater fraternization and exchange of thought between the two professions of law and medicine. While many have worked on interdisciplinary codes at the state level, there is a need for this fraternization in learned societies and in programs conducted at the national and local level.

12. There is a continuing need for lawyers to acquaint physicians with the goals or methods of the adversary system. There is likewise a need for the pertinent and authoritative medical literature of the case to be mobilized. The medical practitioner may not have time to prepare an exhaustive medical brief. The fee of the able advocate may warrant his assuming responsibility for making this search. The responsibility for saying what may constitute valid criteria of proof, however, belongs to the medical profession. Systematic research and teaching are obvious solutions to the problem.

13. Trial lawyers must be considerate of the physician who is earnestly striving to give objective testimony. Firm cross-examination, proceeding from authoritative medical articles, should be courteous. Disagreement based upon strong contradictory evidence is often preferable to a frontal attack that is so severe that the physician may be humiliated so that he defensively resolves never again to lend his efforts to the quest for justice.

INDEX

A

Adrenalectomy, 3, 10
Anguish, 186
Anticonvulsants
   Dilantin, 46, 47, 65
   potassium bromide, 47
   Tegretal, 47
   Tolseram, 47

C

Cancer
   breast, 3, 10
   cordotomy in, 27, 35
   pelvic, 22
   trigeminal tractotomy in, 72
Catabolite, 153
Central pain, 95, 119, 138
Compression
   facial, 64
   trigeminal, 47
Convulsion, *see* Epilepsy
Cordotomy, 25, 33, 89
Cryoprobe, 11

D

Deafferentiation, 53, 59, 64, 129

E

Elavil (or Triavil), 22, 51, 72
Epilepsy, 47, 52, 64, 95-117, 119-136

G

"Gate" theory, 51, 150, 169

H

Hemifacial spasm, 64, 108
Hypophysectomy, 10, 88

I

Ischemic pain, 154

L

Legal aspects, 186
Level of demarcation, 128
Linguistic parallelism, 179

M

Modality (pain), 58, 138, 168
Multiple sclerosis, 50
Muscle pain, 154

N

Nervus intermedius, 64
Neuralgia
   other, 51, 53, 95
   post herpetic, 51, 119
   trigeminal, 42, 47, 75, 76, 119

O

Ovaries, 3

P

Pantopaque, 25
Percodan, 22, 72
Pituitary, 3, 10

R

Rhizotomy
   sacral, 20
   trigeminal, 42

S

Seizure, *see* Epilepsy
Stereotaxic
   cordotomy, 33
   hypophysectomy, 10
   midbrain, 95
   thalamus, 81, 95
   tractotomy, trigeminal, 69
Strategies and tactics in treatment, 176
Summation, 58, 113, 138-152, 164

T

Thinking about pain, 176
Tic douloureux, *see* Neuralgia, trigeminal
Tractotomy, trigeminal, 69

X

X-ray convergence, 86